1   IN THE UNITED STATES COURT OF FEDERAL

2   CLAIMS

3   OFFICE OF SPECIAL MASTERS

4

5   MARK MILES, legal   )

6   representative of a minor   )

7   child, J.M.,   )

8   Petitioner,   ) Case No. 12-254V

9   vs.   )

10 SECRETARY OF HEALTH AND HUMAN)

11 SERVICES,   )

12   Respondent.   )

13 _____)

14

15   OSM ANNEX

16   1401 H STREET, NW

17   WASHINGTON, D.C.

18   WEDNESDAY, OCTOBER 18, 2017

19   9:40 A.M.

20

21   BEFORE SPECIAL MASTER LAURA D. MILLMAN

1

2   REPORTED BY: KRISTY L. CLARK, RPR, NV CCR #708,

3   CA CSR #13529

4

5

```
1    APPEARANCES:

2    For the Petitioner:

3                    JOHN F. MCHUGH, ESQ.

4                    JOHN F. MCHUGH, PC

5                    233 Broadway

6                    Suite 2320

7                    New York, New York 10279

8                    (212) 483-0875

9                    jfmchughpc@aol.com

10

11   For the Respondent:

12

13                   DARRYL R. WISHARD, ESQ.

14                   SHARON SOANES, ESQ.

15                   U.S. DEPARTMENT OF JUSTICE

16                   TORTS BRANCH, CIVIL DIVISION

17                   P.O. Box 146

18                   Benjamin Franklin Station

19                   Washington, D.C. 20044-1046

20                   (202) 616-4357

21                   darryl.wishard@usdoj.gov

22
```

1

2

3

4

```
1                  P R O C E E D I N G S

2                    *  *  *  *  *  *  *

3                 (Proceedings called to order,

4  9:40 a.m.)

5

6

7                 SPECIAL MASTER MILLMAN:  We are on the

8    record.  This is our second day of hearing.  And

9    respondent's counsel has provided me with what

10   respondent will file as Exhibit T, and

11 petitioner's

12   counsel has advised me that they also have the

13 same

14   information but in a official form from the

15 government,

16   but it contains exactly the same.

17                 And what we're going to focus on are

18 on the

19   prior flu vaccinations that we know of that JM

20   took in 2006 and 2008.  There is a reference to

21 the
```

1   2004 vaccination which we discussed later in the

2   afternoon yesterday which Mr. Miles said that JM

3   had received because he had a fever of 101 to

4 103

5   within 24. And the nurse wrote CX on the bottom

6 of the

7   sheet, which was Exhibit 1 at page 63 which

8 means

9   canceled, and she canceled, no doubt because he

10 had a

11   fever beforehand and she wasn't going to

12 inoculate him.

13   There is a reference in there also

14 that

15   before 2004, JM had received other flu

16   vaccinations, but we had no record of that, and

1   respondent as well, and I'm sure respondent is

2   accurate

3   about that.

4   So the reason we're putting Dr.

5   Bellanti back

6   on the stand, and you're still under oath, is to

7   flesh

8   out a little bit more of his testimony

9   yesterday, and

10 it's also in his expert report, that the reason

11 that

12 JM had a reaction within a day, and it is within

13 a

14 day, because of his vaccinations -- sorry,

15 vaccination

16 was October 1st, 2009, between 3:30 and 4:00

17 p.m., and

18 the next, whenever the father could tell us what

19 time

20 of day it was that he did the urine dipstick

21 test, had

1   plus three protein. It could be less than a day

2   depending on what time of day that was. That's

3 short.

4   But -- Doctor -- as an interval.

5   But Dr. Bellanti said, well, there's

6 an

7   anamnestic response because he had flu vaccine

8 at least

9   in 2008. We can see from 2006, which is in

10 Exhibit T,

11   that the components of that -- now, I'm not

12 telling

13   Dr. Bellanti to say there's no anamnestic

14 response due

15   to, because I noticed, however, that none of the

16   components, there's three, of the 2006 flu

17 vaccination

18   are included in the 2008 vaccination or the 2009

19   vaccination. And we're talking about October

20 1st,

21   2009.

1   We can see from Exhibit 1 and 3,

2 November 19,

1   2008, trivalent influenza vaccine used in the

2 2008 to

3   2009 flu season included A/Brisbane/59/2007

4 which is an

5   H1N1-like virus. The second viral strain was

6   A/Brisbane/10/2007 which is an H3N2-like virus.

7 And

8   B/Florida/4/2006-like virus.

9   The October 1st, 2009, trivalent flu

10 vaccine

11   use in the 2009 and 2010 flu season, reference

12   Exhibit 16 and 23, included the same first two

13   components, but not the third one, the first

14 being

15   A/Brisbane/59/2007, H1N1-like virus. The second

16   component being A/Brisbane/10/2007, H3N2-like

17 virus.

18   The third, which is different than the 2008

19 virus --

20   vaccine, was B/Brisbane/60/2008-like virus.

21   So, Dr. Bellanti --

1   MR. WISHARD: Ma'am.

2   SPECIAL MASTER MILLMAN: Yes, Mr.

3 Wishard.

4   MR. WISHARD: There is a discrepancy

5 between

6   that slide and what I have on Exhibit T for the

7 virus.

8   That says that B/Uruguay/716/2007. The

9 information I

10   got from my client was the B/Brisbane/60/2008.

11 I don't

12   know if that makes any difference, but I -- I

13 just want

14   to raise that before --

15   SPECIAL MASTER MILLMAN: Well, thank

16 you for

17   calling my attention to that. Yes, we have a

18 slide

19   from Mr. Miles' computer, and we're going to get

20 a hard

1   copy of that filed. But right now, we're just

2 relying

3   on the slide.

4   It is consistent with the 2008 viral

5   components, but it is not consistent with the

6 2009

7   viral components only in the sense that the

8 third

9   component, instead of what Mr. Wishard got from

10 HHS --

11   Was it HHS?

12   MR. WISHARD: Yes, ma'am.

13   SPECIAL MASTER MILLMAN: Yeah.

14   B/Brisbane/60/2008-like virus,

15 according to

16   the visual representation on the screen is not

17 that,

18   but B/Uruguay/716/2007.

19   THE WITNESS: Yeah. That should be

20   B/Florida/04/2006.

21   SPECIAL MASTER MILLMAN: I'm sorry?

1   THE WITNESS: That vaccine that was

2 received

3   on the -- October the 1st, the B strain is

4   B/Florida/04/2006.   We were having a little

5 trouble --

6   MR. MILES: I think she's talking

7 about the

8   2009.   There were a couple of different Bs that

9 were

10   used in 2009.

11   SPECIAL MASTER MILLMAN: Okay.   And

12 how do

13   you know which one was used if you have a couple

14 of

15   different?

16   MR. MILES: I pulled it up off the --

17 I'm

1   sure they probably pulled it the same place, but

2   it's -- in the product information, there are a

3 couple

4   of different strains that were used. And if you

5 go to

6   the World Health Organization, they have a

7 couple of

8   strains that were listed.

9   SPECIAL MASTER MILLMAN: Okay.

10   MR. MILES: I believe that when he has

11 Uruguay, I can't tell you for sure because I'd

12 have to

13 contact the manufacturer and get that lot and

14 match

15 that up.

16   SPECIAL MASTER MILLMAN: It may not be

17 by

18 lot. It may be -- you know, the flu vaccine, I

19 don't

20 know -- the World Health Organization is the

21 world.

1   MR. MILES: The -- the lot -- the lot

2 would

3   tell.

4   SPECIAL MASTER MILLMAN: It's not just

5 the

6   United States. Mr. Wishard's source is HHS.

7 And CDC

8   is part of HHS. I couldn't speak about more on

9 the

10   authenticity of it or not. It may make

11 absolutely no

12   difference to Dr. Bellanti's testimony because

13 we all

14   know the third component is different in 2009

15 than it

16   was in 2008.

17   MR. MILES: It was not. It was not.

18   SPECIAL MASTER MILLMAN: So whether

19 it's

20   B/Uruguay/716/2007 or B/Brisbane/60/2008, it may

21 make

1   no difference to him.

2   MR. MILES: And just a matching on the

3   -- the

4   two A strains on both years are exactly the

5   same, but

6   the B strains were different; correct.

7   SPECIAL MASTER MILLMAN: Well, we've

8   all said

9   that. I've said it three times.

10   THE WITNESS: Yes.

11   SPECIAL MASTER MILLMAN: All right.

12 So,

13 Mr. McHugh, you're standing at the podium, did

14 you want

15 to ask the question or do you want me to ask the

16 question? It makes no difference to me.

17   MR. McHUGH: I'll defer to you, Your

18 Honor.

19   SPECIAL MASTER MILLMAN: Okay.

20 Doctor,

21 yesterday you were talking, and it's in your

1 reports,

2　expert reports as well, that one of the reasons

3 or

4　maybe the only reason, I can't remember if it's

5 the

6　only one, that you would say this one or maybe

7 less

8　than one day onset if you completely eliminated

9 the

10　5-pound weight gain between September 30th,

11 2009, and

12　October 1st, 2009, and say it's irrelevant

13 because a

14　nephrologist is going to look for spilling of

15 protein.

16　They're not going to look at weight gain.

17 Weight gain

18　is irrelevant except we can see that the rest of

19 the

20　month he kept gaining weight and he wasn't

21 putting on

1   more clothes. So I leave that up to the

2 nephrologist.

1   But you said, relying upon -- let's

2 look at

3   the protein. That's what's important. Weight

4 gain,

5   eh, who knows. That -- that fast response, if

6 it is a

7   response, on October 2nd, the day after the

8   vaccination, is due to an anamnestic response,

9 it's

10   like challenge, rechallenge. When you're

11 exposed to

12   the same substance that you have some kind of

13   sensitivity to, the next time you're exposed to

14 it,

15   you're more sensitive and the third time you

16 die.

17   So have I expressed that correctly?

18   THE WITNESS: Yes, you have, Your

19 Honor. But

20   in addition to what -- in addition to the

21 anamnestic

1   response which would explain a shorter time of

2 the

3   adaptive immune system being stimulated, you

4 have the

5   component of the innate system being stimulated

6 which

7   contributes to more immediacy of the reaction

8 occurring

9   on the 2nd of October. So yes, it is the

10 anamnestic

11   response of the adaptive immune response as well

12 as the

13   contribution of innate stimulation. And I had

14 several

15   references to cytokines that are produced in

16 that

17   particular period that could contribute to the

18 damage

19   that is part of the nephrotic syndrome relapse.

20   SPECIAL MASTER MILLMAN: Clarify for

21 me, if

1   you would, in my mind, which could be totally

2 wrong, I

3   think of it -- an innate response, which is of

4 course

1   very quick, as an allergic response, whereas the

2   adaptive response is more of the immune mediated

3   response; is that correct?

4   THE WITNESS: Adaptive immune, yes.

5   SPECIAL MASTER MILLMAN: So is it your

6   testimony that JM had an allergic response which

7   is why he had spillage of protein plus three the

8 day

9   after his flu vaccination of October 1st, 2009?

10   THE WITNESS: Yes. Well, it's not

11 allergic

12   in the sense of the usual allergies, the IGE.

13 It's not

14   that kind of a response. But it is a

15 hypersensitivity

16   response.

17   And I think if you could show -- if

18 you could

19   just show that innate slide, if you go down a

20 few.

21   Just go down quickly, please. It shows the --

1 where

2   the innate system comes in and where the

3 adaptive

4   system comes in.

5   Keep going, please. That one.

6   You see schematically, this slide

7 shows the

8   innate immunity being stimulated within minutes,

9 hours,

10   or even a few days, whereas the adaptive takes a

11 little

12   longer. But with the anamnestic response, it's

13 even

14   pushed more to the left. So you have the

15 anamnestic

16   response of the adaptive immunity plus the

17 contribution

18   of the innate immunity. And this has now been

1   referenced in several of the articles that I

2 submitted,

3   particularly the Koenig article from the FDA,

4   indicating that the innate system has to be

5 looked at

6   in addition to this anamnestic adaptive.

7   So both are operative, Your Honor.

8   SPECIAL MASTER MILLMAN: Thank you.

9 Thank

10   you for the clarification.

11   Now, let me ask you the question that

12 was,

13   I'm sure, Mr. McHugh's only question for you,

14 which is:

15   Now that you know the components of the 2008 --

16 well,

17   you actually also know 2006, but it seems

18 irrelevant

19   unless you think it's relevant, which you have

20 to tell

21   me. But I would think that you're going to

1 focus on

2   2008-2009.

3   Can you explain that?

4   THE WITNESS: Yes. Could we go back

5 to that

6   slide, please, the third slide.

7   I wanted to clarify, Your Honor,

8 something

9   that the respondent's lawyers were -- were

10 pursuing

11   with me. And we wanted to clarify this issue of

12 the

13   2004 immunization that I was pressed to admit to

14 based

15   upon the record that was provided to me. In

16 fact, the

17   record that was provided to me is incorrect.

18 And I

19   refer you to Exhibit --

20   SPECIAL MASTER MILLMAN: Pardon me?

1   MR. McHUGH: Exhibit 1-63.

2   THE WITNESS: I refer you to Exhibit

3 1,

4   page 63 --

5   SPECIAL MASTER MILLMAN: Yes.

6   THE WITNESS: -- which is entitled

7 "The

8   Willow Bend Pediatrics Report," from the office

9 of

10   Michael Frank. And I will -- the -- the

11 respondent's

12   were pressing me on the statement that a vaccine

13 given

14   in the left thigh on Lot U1417AA, expiration

15 date

16   6/3/05, NDC492837415, was actually given. And

17 we had a

18   lengthy discussion, you may recall, because one

19 of the

20   items suggested in this protocol was does the

21 patient

1   have an allergy to eggs and chicken?   No.   Has

2 the

3   patient had a fever greater than 101 in the past

4   24 hours?   And it was checked yes.

5   So based upon that, we would have

6 assumed

7   that the patient didn't receive it.   But there

8 was a

9   discrepancy.   It's -- it looked like they

10 indicated a

11   vaccine had been given, but then at the bottom

12 of the

13   page, there's a star which said the patient had

14 a

15   temperature of 101 to 103 within the past 24

16 hours, and

17   then the acronym CX.

18   Now, that was a mystery for a while

19 until

20   Mr. Miles called the nurse who actually

21 annotated that.

1   And CX in their terminology -- I never use

2 acronyms --

1   means canceled. So in fact, the truth is that

2   this

3   patient did not receive the vaccine in 2004.

4   So I wanted that to be clarified.

5   This is

6   the truth.

7   BY MR. McHUGH:

8   Q.   Okay. Doctor, let's -- can you get --

9   A.   So the actual vaccines that this child

10 received, the three vaccines that are related to

11 influenza, are on this slide which includes the

12 live

13 attenuated vaccine on November the 20th of 2006.

14 Second vaccine, inactivated influenza vaccine,

15 on

16 November the 19th on 2008, and the third vaccine

17 which

18 was the putative vaccine that caused this

19 relapse of

20 nephrotic syndrome was given, is another

21 inactivated

1   vaccine. And the conscriptions and the content

2 of

3   these are exactly, Your Honor, as you indicated.

4 Both

5   of those -- well, the third -- they all are

6 similar.

7   They have the H1N1, the H3N2 A viruses, and the

8   -- a

9   third would be the B. And so these are the

10 actual only

11 three vaccines that this child received. So I

12 wanted

13 to clarify that for the record.

14   SPECIAL MASTER MILLMAN: It's not

15 actually

16 true that he only received these three flu

17 vaccinations

18 because we know from Exhibit 1, page 63, that

19 the nurse

20 had circled, probably because Mr. Miles answered

21 her

1   question, that before 2004, JM had received flu

2   vaccinations. Because the first question is:

3   Is this

4   the first influenza vaccine this child has

5   received?

6   And it was no.

7   THE WITNESS: Yes, I refer you to

8   Exhibit 12

9   page 2, Your Honor. And this is a complete

10 listing of

11   all the vaccines that were given at the Willow

12 Bend

13   Pediatrics. Beginning in 2001, DPTs, tetanus,

14 HIV,

15   inactivated polio vaccine, MMR, the pneumococcal

16   vaccines, the varicella vaccine, and that is a

17 complete

18   list. And the only ones that relate to the

19   influenza --

20   MR. WISHARD: Excuse me, ma'am.

21   THE WITNESS: -- are those that we

1 mentioned.

2   SPECIAL MASTER MILLMAN: Okay. I'm on

3 12.

4   MR. WISHARD: I'm trying to move to

5 where

6   they're at. I'm not sure where we're at.

7   SPECIAL MASTER MILLMAN: I'm sorry.

8 I'm

9   missing things when people talk over each other,

10 and

11   whoever's unfortunate to have to transcribe this

12 is

13   going to say, what?

14   MR. WISHARD: Sorry.

15   SPECIAL MASTER MILLMAN: So all right.

16 We'll

17   start with Mr. Wishard, and then Mr. McHugh can

18 say

19   whatever he wants.

1   Mr. Wishard, what?

2   MR. WISHARD: I was just wanting to

3 know what

4 Dr. Bellanti was reading, what exhibit and page

5 number.

6   SPECIAL MASTER MILLMAN: It was

7 Exhibit 12.

8   THE WITNESS: I'm sorry. Exhibit 12.

9   SPECIAL MASTER MILLMAN: Page 1.

10   THE WITNESS: Page 1.

11   SPECIAL MASTER MILLMAN: That's what

12 I'm

13 looking at right now.

14   MR. McHUGH: It's actually page 2 and

15 3.

16   MR. WISHARD: Thank you.

17   SPECIAL MASTER MILLMAN: What about

18 page 2

19 and 3?

20   MR. McHUGH: Page 2 and 3. Exhibit

21 12,

1   page 2 and 3.

2   SPECIAL MASTER MILLMAN: From my

3 notes, I

4 only ran off page 1. Okay. So --

5 BY MR. McHUGH:

6   Q.   So, in other words, Doctor, there is

7 no

8 official record of any other -- any other flu

9 vaccine

10   other than these.

11   A.   Other than the ones that we spoke of,

12 that is

13 correct, Mr. McHugh.

14   SPECIAL MASTER MILLMAN: One moment,

15 please.

16   We're not moving on yet. Okay. I don't have 2

17 and 3

1   in front of me because I only ran off page 1.

2   MR. McHUGH: Okay. Let me give you --

3   MR. WISHARD: I have it up if you want

4 to --

5   SPECIAL MASTER MILLMAN: Sure.

6   MR. WISHARD: -- just if he wants to

7 put it

8   up on the big screen, I have it up on my

9 computer.

10   SPECIAL MASTER MILLMAN: Thank you.

11   MR. WISHARD: There's 3, and this is

12 3,

13   ma'am, just so you know. I don't know where you

14 want

15   me to go.

16   SPECIAL MASTER MILLMAN: Thank you.

17   So this is 2?

18   MR. WISHARD: Yes, ma'am.

19   SPECIAL MASTER MILLMAN: Okay.

20   MR. WISHARD: I can make it bigger if

21 you

1   need me to make it bigger.

2   SPECIAL MASTER MILLMAN: I'm trying to

3 figure

4   out what in heaven's name -- oh, there they are.

5 If --

6   okay.

7   If you could scroll up a little bit.

8   MR. WISHARD: Yes, ma'am.

9   SPECIAL MASTER MILLMAN: No.   I mean

10 the

11   other way.   Thank you.

12   MR. McHUGH: It's the next page is the

13 flu

14   vaccine.

1   SPECIAL MASTER MILLMAN: All right.

2 Okay.

3   Stop. Okay. You've got 2006 for FluMist. So

4   according to this record, the 2006 vaccination

5 wasn't

6   inactivated. It -- but we already knew that.

7 It was

8   FluMist. And go down to the rest of the page.

9 So it

10   doesn't include what we're talking about.

11   This is not a complete record because

12 it

13   omits -- I know he switched -- probably

14 switched.

15   THE WITNESS: Well, this record was

16 dated --

17   I'm sorry.

18   Do you have a date on that? Eight --

19   MR. WISHARD: I don't know which date

20 you

21   want. Down here?

1   THE WITNESS: Birth date was given,

2 but the

3   date of the recording might not have

4 encapsulated the

5   more recent influenza.

6   SPECIAL MASTER MILLMAN: Okay. Now,

7 we have

8   Mr. Miles here, and Mr. Miles is near a

9 microphone and

10 Mr. Miles told me yesterday --

11   MR. MILES: Yes, ma'am.

12   SPECIAL MASTER MILLMAN: -- when we

13 were off

14 the record that he was present when the nurse

15 was

16 writing all these answers down because she

17 wouldn't

18 have known unless somebody told her.

19   MR. MILES: I don't believe she

20 questioned

1   it. It looks like a premade form and she

2   probably

3   filled it out before she even came in and then

4   she

5   circles --

6   SPECIAL MASTER MILLMAN: Wait a

7   minute. I

8   didn't follow that at all.

9   MR. MILES: In terms of the circling,

10 she's

11 assuming, probably from the records, that he's

12 had it

13 before. I don't think she actually filled it

14 out

15 properly or asked me any questions on that.

16   SPECIAL MASTER MILLMAN: Well, how

17 would she

18 have known he had a fever?

19   MR. MILES: Because they tested him

20 for a

21 fever when he first walked in terms --

1   SPECIAL MASTER MILLMAN: So she filled

2 out

3   that whole form by herself and never asked

4 either you

5   or your wife any questions?

6   MR. MILES: The lot. Everything's

7 already

8   filled in, yes. And she probably just made

9 assumptions

10   that he's had it before. And then technically,

11 if she

12   checked the records, she would know that he

13 never had

14   it. If you go from 2008 and 2012, I got letters

15 from

16   the doctor. That should be in the record. I'm

17 not

18   sure where, what exhibit. I can give it to you

19 right

20   here. I highlighted it.

21   SPECIAL MASTER MILLMAN: What?

1   MR. MILES: In both instances, they

2 were done

3   by Dr. Seikaly at Children's Medical Center.

4   SPECIAL MASTER MILLMAN: You mean the

5 2008

6   and 2009?

7   MR. MILES: Correct.

8   SPECIAL MASTER MILLMAN: What about

9 2006?

10   Oh, that's --

11   MR. MILES: 2006 was done by Dr.

12 Frank.

13   SPECIAL MASTER MILLMAN: Okay. Is it

14 your

15   testimony, and you're still under oath --

16   MR. MILES: Yes.

17   SPECIAL MASTER MILLMAN: -- that JM

18   never received a flu vaccination until November

19 20,

20   2006?

21   MR. MILES: Correct.

1   SPECIAL MASTER MILLMAN: Okay.   That

2   clarifies that.

3   THE WITNESS: Okay, Your Honor.

4   SPECIAL MASTER MILLMAN: We have no

5 proof

6   otherwise.   I don't know how else you're going

7 to find

8   something different.

9   Yes, Mr. McHugh, I've been keeping you

10   waiting a long time.   What did you want to say?

11   MR. McHUGH: I have only one question

12 left,

13   Your Honor.

1   SPECIAL MASTER MILLMAN: Okay. So let

2 me

3   return to Dr. Bellanti. We keep moving away

4 from this

5   back and forth and back and forth. It's kind of

6 like

7   watching waves coming in and going out.

8   Is it your testimony that having two

9 out of

10   three components that are the same between 2008

11 and

12   2009 is sufficient immunological identification

13 so that

14   JM would have an anamnestic response the day

15 after

16   his October 1st, 2009, vaccine?

17   THE WITNESS: Yes. Yes, your Honor.

18   SPECIAL MASTER MILLMAN: It is. Okay.

19 You

20   have to educate me a little bit.

21   We're all familiar with people who are

1   allergic to peanuts, and sometimes you read this

2 really

3   awful short newspaper article about the girl

4 who's

5   allergic to peanuts and her mother never gives

6 her

7   anything that has peanuts in it, is very

8 vigilant

9   because it's so bad. And she and her girlfriend

10 are in

11   elementary school and they open up their lunch

12 and

13   their friend's lunch has peanuts. And just the

14 odor of

15   the peanuts --

16   THE WITNESS: Yes.

17   SPECIAL MASTER MILLMAN: -- she

18 collapses and

19   she dies.

20   THE WITNESS: Yes. Yes.

1   SPECIAL MASTER MILLMAN: Right. Okay.

2 But

3   that's peanuts. Peanuts, peanuts, peanuts.

4   And one of the articles that you

5 submitted

6   about an adult who had, I don't know, nephrotic

7   syndrome after her third hepatitis B

8 vaccination,

9   excuse me, Mr. Wishard I think it was, maybe it

10 was

11   Ms. Soanes, I don't remember, said, But that's

12 the same

13   vaccine. It's identical. Hepatitis 1,

14 hepatitis 2,

15   hepatitis 3, all B vaccine. They're identical.

16   This is not identical. And, of

17 course, it's

18   not given in the sequence. You -- you give

19 hepatitis B

20   vaccine in Series 1, 2, and 3 within three or

21 four

1   months. Here you've got a year between November

2   19th,

3   2008, and October 1st, 2009.

4   Is an anamnestic response going to

5   happen --

6   THE WITNESS: Yes.

7   SPECIAL MASTER MILLMAN: -- in that

8   length of

9   time --

10   THE WITNESS: Yes.

11   SPECIAL MASTER MILLMAN: -- when

12   there's

13   some -- something different about the

14   ingredients or

15   something or other?

16   THE WITNESS: Yes. The immunological

17   memory

18   is encapsulated in the T and the B cells. And

19   you may

20   recall the discussion we had about the swine flu

21   and

1   those older patients who had experienced the --

2   the

3   famous Spanish influenza in 1918 still retain

4   memory

5   cells in their blood that responded to the new

6   swine

7   flu. There was some cross-reactivity. Excuse

8   me.

9   SPECIAL MASTER MILLMAN: Don't hit the

10   microphone.

11   THE WITNESS: There was some cross-

12   reactivity

13   between the swine flu influenza and the 1918

14   strain.

15   So this immunologic memory lasts a long time.

16 And I

17   think there's definitely enough evidence to

18 support

19   immunologic memory based upon the live

20 attenuated given

21   in 2006 and the two -- the previous 2008

1 inactivated

2 vaccine to stimulate an anamnestic response.

3   SPECIAL MASTER MILLMAN: All right.

4 We have

5 one identical component -- no, I'm sorry. I'm

6 looking

7 at the wrong vaccine. We don't have any

8 identical

9 component between the 2006 and the 2008 or

10 between the

11 2006 and the 2009.

12   So why would the 2006 be relevant at

13 all?

14   THE WITNESS: You know, the story with

15 influenza, Your Honor, and I've had an

16 opportunity to

17 study this when I was at Walter Reed Army

18 Institute of

19 Research. Tommy Francis, Dr. Francis, in

20 Michigan

21 and -- and those workers with influenza vaccine,

1 spoke

2   about original -- they called it original

3 immunologic

1   sin that was imprinted the first time you're

2 exposed.

3   Every time you're exposed to new viruses that

4 there is

5   some molecular mimicry, if you will, some

6   cross-reactivity, it's enough to give you that

7   anamnestic response. There's sharing of these

8   epitopes, so that, you know, whether we're

9 talking

10   about Brisbane or Australia or Uruguay or

11 Florida,

12   there's enough similarity with those antigenic

13 epitopes

14   to stimulate the anamnestic response.

15   SPECIAL MASTER MILLMAN: So is it your

16   testimony that the fact that you've got two A

17 flu

18   strains and one B flu strain is sufficient

19 identity --

20   THE WITNESS: Yes.

21   SPECIAL MASTER MILLMAN: -- among

1 2006, 2008,

2   and 2009 that there would be this anamnestic

3 response

4   in 2009 based on the prior two vaccines?

5   THE WITNESS: That's correct.

6   SPECIAL MASTER MILLMAN: What do you

7 mean by

8   cross-reactivity?

9   THE WITNESS: I'm sorry?

10   SPECIAL MASTER MILLMAN: You mentioned

11 in the

12   context of swine flu vaccine program 1976, that

13 there

14   were people who were alive in 1918 that had been

15   exposed but didn't die to the pandemic 1918 flu

16   epidemic which actually killed mostly young

17 people in

1   their 20s.

2   THE WITNESS: Yes.

3   SPECIAL MASTER MILLMAN: And that

4 created a

5   cross-reactivity when they received the 1976 flu

6   vaccination.

7   What does that mean, cross-reactivity?

8   THE WITNESS: What does it mean in

9 terms of?

10   SPECIAL MASTER MILLMAN: No. You --

11 you said

12   they discovered they had -- discovered

13   cross-reactivity. I don't know what you're

14 talking

15   about.

16   THE WITNESS: What this means is that

17 those

18   older individuals who were still living in 1976

19 had

20   sufficient memory, immunologic memory so that if

21 they

1   were exposed to this swine flu, which never

2   turned out

3   to be an epidemic of course, they would have

4   been

5   stimulated, would have been protected. They

6   would not

7   have developed the disease. The antibody that

8   would be

9   stimulated is protective, protective antibody.

10 So

11 that -- I was just using that as an example of

12 sharing

13 of antigens.

14   SPECIAL MASTER MILLMAN: I do hate

15 mathematics, but maybe we could work this out

16 together.

17 If somebody were alive in 1918 to be exposed to

18 that

19 pandemic flu virus, of course we have to make up

20 this

1   person right now, how old would that person be

2 in 1976?

3   THE WITNESS: Well, if you were 18 in

4 1918 --

5   SPECIAL MASTER MILLMAN: You'd be 76.

6   THE WITNESS: -- you would be 76.

7   SPECIAL MASTER MILLMAN: I could do

8 that. I

9   can do that. Oh, very good. Okay.

10   This brings you back to the question

11 you

12   couldn't answer yesterday: Why are people, the

13   elderly, there are at least a few of us in this

14 room,

15   why are the elderly encouraged to a get a high-

16 dose flu

17   vaccination when they've been exposed to either

18 flu

19   vaccines for 55 years or the actual flu itself?

20 They

21   should be immune. They don't need anything.

1   THE WITNESS: Exactly.   That's a very

2 good

3   question, Your Honor.   If I can draw a circle

4 and then

5   an inner circle, and let's say the outer circle

6 are the

7   memory cells and the inner circle are the new

8 cells

9   that are going to be stimulated again.   If you

10 compare

11   an infant with an elderly person the circles are

12 like

13   this (witness indicating).   In the infant, the

14 outer

15   circle -- or the inner circle is huge.   They've

16 got a

17   great --

18   SPECIAL MASTER MILLMAN: Because they

19 have no

20   memory cells.

21   THE WITNESS: They've got potential

1 memory

1   cells but few actual memory cells. In the

2 adult, the

3   circle, the inner circle, their ability to make

4 new

5   responses to an antigen-like influence is very

6 small.

7   So you really have to stimulate it with a high

8 dose

9   because unlike a younger infant who has the

10 greater

11   capacity of making new memory cells, the elderly

12 don't

13   have that. That's why we use the high dose.

14   SPECIAL MASTER MILLMAN: I have

15 another

16   question for you. You know that there's a

17 shingles

18   vaccine --

19   THE WITNESS: Yes.

20   SPECIAL MASTER MILLMAN: -- Zostavax,

21   Z-o-s-t-a-v-a-x, and it is really like varicella

1   vaccine --

2   THE WITNESS: It is.

3   SPECIAL MASTER MILLMAN: -- except

4 it's

5   ramped up. I forget how many more antigens are

6 in it

7   than what children would get in school. And

8 that is to

9   prevent shingles, because once you have been

10 exposed to

11   chickenpox, as those of us of a certain age

12 have, it

13   doesn't go away. It lurks in your spinal cord.

14 And at

15   some point, you might get shingles. That is to

16 protect

17   you.

18   Well, if you have all these wonderful

19 memory

20   cells, why wouldn't you be protected? Why would

21 you

1   needs Zostavax?

2   THE WITNESS: Okay. That's another

3 good

4   question, Your Honor. There's a misconception,

5   actually, and there's very few people that

6 understand

7   this. And I was fortunate to have worked with

8 people

9   that -- and we did some of our research in

10 what's

11   called cell-mediated immunity. The immune

12 system of

13   the adaptive system consists of the T cells and

14 the

15   B cells, as I showed yesterday. The B cells

16 make

17   antibody. The T cells do a lot of things. They

18 help

19   B cells. They do this. They do that. They

20 send --

21   there's a lot of functions.

```
 1              When you get chickenpox as a child,

 2  unlike

 3   viruses like the common cold and influenza that

 4  goes

 5   away when you are clearing it, these viruses,

 6  the

 7   herpes viruses have a propensity to become

 8  latent.

 9   They never go away.  They stay in those cells

10  that you

11   refer to in -- along the spinal canal.  And

12  they're

13   kept in check by the T cells not the B cells.

14              And when you're stressed, you know,

15  with

16   steroids or with stress or with any kind of

17  infection,

18   when the T cells lose their function, out comes

19  the

20   sleeping giant, and that virus then follows a

21  nerve
```

1   rootlet in what we call shingles.   So the idea

2 of

3   giving a vaccine to adults over 60 or 65 is to

1   stimulate the T cells not the B cells.

2   Actually, if you look at the serum of

3 these

4   elderly people, they have plenty of antibody,

5 but it's

6   doing no good because the virus is in the cells.

7 You

8   have to keep the T cells up. And that's what

9 the

10   studies of Levine did in the University of

11 Maryland

12   many years ago. He showed that when you give

13 the

14   vaccine, you're stimulating the T cells. So

15 that's why

16   there's a discrepancy, and understanding

17 actually,

18   about this. But that's -- that's why we give

19 the

20   vaccine.

21   SPECIAL MASTER MILLMAN: All right.

1   JM's onset of his nephrotic syndrome was 2007,

2 if

3   I remember correctly.

4   THE WITNESS: The first one, yes,

5 2007.

6   SPECIAL MASTER MILLMAN: Okay.

7   THE WITNESS: Could we show that

8 timeline,

9   the third slide, please.

10   SPECIAL MASTER MILLMAN: Oh, thank

11 you. I

12   don't know how you find one slide from another.

13   THE WITNESS: Yes, it was 2007.

14   SPECIAL MASTER MILLMAN: Okay. Thank

15 you.

16   THE WITNESS: And on the slide, it

17 would be

18   indicated in the center of the slide on

19 10/1/2009. And

20   in yellow we see the flu vaccine being given,

21 and

1   that's that third vaccine that we were talking

2   about.

3   SPECIAL MASTER MILLMAN: I see lots of

4   yellows. Where? Oh, okay. I got you.

5   This is my question: He goes into

6   remission -- and thank you for the slide. He

7   goes into

8   remission in August 2008; is that correct? It's

9   on the

10   left.

11   THE WITNESS: Yes. Yes, the first

12   highlight.

13   SPECIAL MASTER MILLMAN: Thank you.

14   He gets vaccinated against flu vaccine

15   November 19th, 2008. That's his second flu

16   vaccine.

17   The first one was November 20th, 2006, before he

18   ever

19   came down --

20   THE WITNESS: Yes.

21   SPECIAL MASTER MILLMAN: -- with

1 nephrotic

2   syndrome.

3   Why, since now there should be an

4 anamnestic

5   effect from the flu vaccination administered

6   November 20, 2006, to the flu vaccination

7 administered

8   November 19th, 2008, didn't he have a relapse

9 then?

10   THE WITNESS: Well, that's a very good

11 question, Your Honor. We obviously don't know

12 the

13 precise answer, but I can offer this based on

14 what we

15 know about these vaccines.

16   First of all -- first of all, the

17 attenuated

1   live influenza vaccine is a subject very dear to

2   my

3   heart because we were the first, actually, to

4   describe

5   the secretory IGA in the nasal secretions

6   following

7   viral infection that offer protection. We made

8   this

9   observation in 1964 with Dr. Ardensene and Dr.

10 Buscher

11 at Walter Reed.

12   The basis for protective immunity when

13 you

14 give a virus intranasally is to stimulate not

15 the

16 IGE -- the IGG but the IGA and the secretions.

17 And

18 the -- our belief and our hope was that these

19 live

20 vaccines like influenza given intranasally would

21 be

1   effective. And we did some studies actually

2 with

3   Dr. Albert Sabin with the measles vaccine given

4   intranasally. And we were hopeful that this was

5 what

6   Dr. Sabin hoped to achieve with nasal vaccines

7 with

8   measles. As it turns out, the influenza, this

9   attenuated vaccine that he received in 2006, is

10 no

11   longer being recommended by the CDC because it

12 doesn't

13   have the punch that we hoped that it would have.

14 So

15   it's not even recommended anymore. It's a great

16   disappointment to me.

17   But to answer your question, it may be

18 that

19   that alone was not sufficient to give enough of

20 an

21   anamnestic response when he received the first

1   inactivated vaccine on 2008.

1   SPECIAL MASTER MILLMAN: So does that

2 mean

3   that the anamnestic effect which you have

4 testified was

5   present in the onset October 2nd, 2009, when he

6 was

7   spilling plus three protein was based, really,

8 only on

9   the November 19th, 2008, kill virus vaccine and

10 not on

11   the November 20th, 2006, attenuated live flu

12 vaccine

13   because that was not efficacious?

14   THE WITNESS: Well, I wouldn't say it

15 was the

16   only. There might have been some response to

17 the

18   attenuated, but it wasn't sufficient enough that

19 giving

20   an inactivated vaccine on 2008 would achieve.

21 So I

1   don't think we could completely eliminate it,

2 but I

3   think the induction of memory cells was largely

4   obtained with that 2008 vaccine given

5 intramuscularly.

6   SPECIAL MASTER MILLMAN: Thank you.

7   In order to have the anamnestic

8 response,

9   would you need to have sensitivity to eggs?

10   THE WITNESS: Oh, no.   No, you would

11 not --

12   in fact, if you're sensitive to eggs, this might

13 --

14   there would be some precaution in giving this

15 vaccine,

16   and there are protocols of how to get around

17 this and

18   study it.   The American Academy of Allergy and

19 the

20   American College of Allergy have guidelines for

21 this.

1   SPECIAL MASTER MILLMAN: Well, we

2 don't know

3   who gave the nurse the information on Exhibit 1,

1   page 63, that JM was not allergic to eggs, but

2   apparently the nurse thought so.

3   THE WITNESS: Yeah, I don't think this

4 is a

5   problem.

6   SPECIAL MASTER MILLMAN: So what is it

7 that

8   your -- when I say "your," I don't mean you, but

9 what

10   is somebody who's experiencing an anamnestic

11 response

12   being sensitized to exactly? If it's not eggs

13 in which

14   the flu vaccine is produced, what -- what is he

15 being

16   sensitized to?

17   THE WITNESS: Well, he's sensitized to

18 the

19   epitopes that are a part of the virus that --

20 this kill

21   virus that's in the vaccine.

1   SPECIAL MASTER MILLMAN: Kind of the

2   fingerprints of the virus?

3   THE WITNESS: Yes, and the

4 fingerprints of

5   the virus. In all of its dimensions, you know,

6 you get

7   this -- it's almost like epitopes spreading that

8 we

9   talk about. Where epitopes cross-react, you get

10   sensitized to one strain. You get another

11 strain, it

12   broadens the spectrum. It's a continuum. And

13 this is

14   what we hope to achieve with influenza. And,

15   unfortunately, it's only what, 50 to 70 percent

16   effective, but it does give some benefit to, you

17 know,

18   denting and blunting the disease.

1   SPECIAL MASTER MILLMAN: I can't

2 remember

3   yesterday as well as I'm sure you do because the

4   -- the

5   question I'm having is dealing with immunology.

6   Dr. Quan mentioned something, I think

7 you

8   mentioned something, and I should look through

9 my

10   notes, but that might take too much time and I

11 might

12   not have written it down too. So let me just

13 ask you

14   if you can recall what I'm trying to remember.

15   There's something about nephrotic

16 syndrome

17   which indicates a lack of immune response or

18 else it's

19   over immune response. That's where I can't

20 remember.

21   Do you recall?

1   THE WITNESS: Well, I think what Dr.

2 Quan

3   was -- was mentioning is that many cases of the

4   nephrotic syndrome are triggered by viruses, the

5 common

6   cold and other respiratory viruses.   I don't

7 recall

8   specifically about too much -- oh, I know what

9 he was

10   referring to.   That -- he was saying that there

11 are

12   clearly immunologic processes that are involved

13 in the

14   pathogenesis of the nephrotic -- of the

15 syndrome.   And

16   when you heighten the immune response in any

17 way, it

18   might throw the balance off for relapse.

19   So he was using that as an example of

20 why,

21   you know, we try to attenuate the immune

1 response.

2   That's why we give steroids, in more serious

3 cases the

1   stronger immunosuppressants. So I think in that

2   context, I think he was referring to too much of

3 an

4   immune response being responsible for the

5 relapse.

6   SPECIAL MASTER MILLMAN: He said

7 something

8   which was very curious, and I'm not going to

9 remember

10   this completely either, but when a child, let's

11 say

12   with minimal change disease, gets measles, the

13 actual

14   disease, they -- this is where I forget -- they

15 either

16   don't or they do get worse. But my recollection

17 is

18   that they actually were better, and it had

19 something to

20   do with T cells.

21   THE WITNESS: Oh, yes, yes. Very

1 good.

2   That's a very good point. This is an

3 observation that

4   was made many, many years ago by a -- one of the

5   founders of allergy. His name was Clemens von

6 Pirquet.

7   SPECIAL MASTER MILLMAN: Do you want

8 to spell

9   that last name for the court reporter.

10   THE WITNESS: Yeah, Clemens, C-l-e-m-

11 o-n-s

12   [sic]. Von Pirquet, V, as in Victor, o-n. Next

13 word,

14   P-i-r-q-u-e-t.

15   SPECIAL MASTER MILLMAN: Thank you.

16   THE WITNESS: He's called the father

17 of

18   allergy actually, but he was a pediatrician

19 involved

20   with infectious diseases. And he observed -- he

21 came

1   from Vienna, Austria, and he was studying

2 infections.

1   And he noted with tuberculosis, many times, you

2 know --

3   well, to this day, we still do skin tests. If

4 you have

5   tuberculosis, you do a skin test which is called

6 a

7   delayed response. Usually, you get a red bump

8 in 24 to

9   48 hours. That means the patient either has or

10 has

11   been exposed to TB.

12   If that patient who has a positive

13 skin test

14   to tuberculin, to tuberculosis is exposed to

15 measles,

16   that goes away. It was an interesting -- and we

17 never

18   understood this for over 100 years. Now, we

19 know that

20   that bouquet of T cells that I was talking about

21   yesterday, the Th1, the Th17, the Th2, and the

1 Treg

2 cells, regulatory cells, those regulatory cells

3 are the

4 ones that silence the immune system. And with

5 measles,

6 those -- there is this disequilibrium that

7 silences the

8 immune response and you get what is called

9 anergy,

10 a-n-e-r-g-y. Hypergy means too much. Anergy,

11 from the

12 Greek, anything with an "a" means too little.

13 You get

14 an anergic response. And we never understood

15 this

16 until the knowledge of the T cells and all the

17 subsets

18 have come in. So that is a -- is an interesting

19 phenomenon. So sometimes infections can

20 actually

21 lessen the immune response. You're right. But

1 for the

2   most part, they would heighten it.

3   SPECIAL MASTER MILLMAN: Thank you.

1   THE WITNESS: That's an interesting

2   observation. But that's -- that's the basis of

3 it.

4   SPECIAL MASTER MILLMAN: All right.

5 Thank

6   you very much.

7   Mr. McHugh, did you have any questions

8 for

9   Dr. Bellanti before I turn him over to Ms.

10 Soanes?

11   MR. McHUGH: I think you've covered

12   everything, Your Honor.

13   SPECIAL MASTER MILLMAN: Oh, so that's

14 a no?

15   MR. McHUGH: That's a no. Thank you.

16   SPECIAL MASTER MILLMAN: You can sit

17 down.

18   Thank you. I'm sorry you were standing so long.

19 I

20   wasn't looking at you. I didn't see. Thank

21 you.

1   Ms. Soanes, did you have any questions

2 on

3   cross?

4   MS. SOANES: No, I do not.

5   SPECIAL MASTER MILLMAN: All right.

6 Thank

7   you, Dr. Bellanti. Appreciate your coming back

8 to the

9   stand. I think Mr. Wishard or Ms. Soanes,

10 whoever's

11 going up first --

12   MR. WISHARD: Petitioner's rest?

13   SPECIAL MASTER MILLMAN: You want to

14 check

15 and make sure?

16   MR. WISHARD: Is that everything?

17   SPECIAL MASTER MILLMAN: You have

18 finished

1   your side except for maybe rebuttal, Mr. McHugh?

2   MR. McHUGH: Yes, petitioner's case is

3   completed.

4   SPECIAL MASTER MILLMAN: Thank you.

5   MR. WISHARD: Call Dr. Kaplan.

6   SPECIAL MASTER MILLMAN: Mr. Wishard.

7   Dr. Kaplan, would you please take the

8   stand.

9   Thank you.

10   MR. WISHARD: Dr. Kaplan, could you

11   please

12   state your name --

13   SPECIAL MASTER MILLMAN: Not yet.

14   Dr. Kaplan, would you raise your right

15   hand,

16   please.

17   Thereupon--

18   BERNARD KAPLAN, M.D.,

19   was called as a witness, and having been first

20   duly

21   sworn, was examined and testified as follows:

343

1

2   THE WITNESS: Yes, I do.

3   SPECIAL MASTER MILLMAN: Would you

4 state your

5   name and professional address for the record,

6 please.

7   THE WITNESS: My name is Bernard

8 Kaplan.

9   Since I'm retired, I have a little room in my

10 house,

11   348 Woodley Road, W-o-o-d-l-e-y, Merion, M-e-r-

12 i-o-n,

13   in Pennsylvania.

1   SPECIAL MASTER MILLMAN: And you have

2 a

3   British accent, do you not?

4   THE WITNESS: I was born as a subject

5 of

6   King George I and subsequently Queen Elizabeth

7 II in

8   South Africa.

9   SPECIAL MASTER MILLMAN: Usually when

10 I ask

11 somebody if they have a British accent, they say

12 I'm

13 from Australia and I never get it straight.

14 Well,

15 welcome to the country.

16   THE WITNESS: Thank you.

17   SPECIAL MASTER MILLMAN: Your witness,

18 Mr. Wishard.

19   MR. WISHARD: Thank you, ma'am.

20

21   DIRECT EXAMINATION

1   BY MR. WISHARD:

2   Q.   You are retired.

3   When did you retire, Dr. Kaplan?

4   A.   I retired officially in June of 2016.

5   Q.   Before you retired, what did you do?

6   A.   Before I retired, I spent eight years

7   at the

8   mercy of the new chief of nephrology, who had me

9   see

10   lots of patients each day in clinic.

11   Q.   And where was that?

12   A.   At the Children's Hospital of

13 Philadelphia.

1   Q.   Since I think this might be the first

2 time

3   you testified in front of special master, I want

4 to go

5   in a little bit about your educational

6 background

7   starting when you were in South Africa.

8   A.   Yes, sir.

9   Q.   Where did you graduate from college?

10   A.   So I graduated from the University of

11   Witwatersrand, W-i-t-w-a-t-e-r -- I told you it

12 was

13   going to be difficult -- r-a-n-d in

14 Johannesburg, South

15   Africa in 1964. And I then spent six months as

16 a

17   surgical intern, six months as a internal

18 medicine

19   intern, and then five and a half years as a

20 pediatric

21   intern and resident in Johannesburg.

1   Subsequent to that, we went to

2   Montreal in

3   Canada where I worked at the children's

4   hospital, the

5   Montreal Children's Hospital as a pediatric --

6   training

7   in pediatric nephrology and at the Royal

8   Victoria

9   Hospital, also in Montreal, training in adults

10   nephrology.

11   After that, I eventually became the

12   director

13   of residency training at McGill University for

14   pediatrics for -- for nine years. And director

15 of the

16   renal laboratory and the renal division, also at

17 the

18   Montreal Children's Hospital. And in 1987, we -

19 -

20   sorry, I keep saying "we."

1   SPECIAL MASTER MILLMAN: Is that the

2 royal we

3   or is that --

4   THE WITNESS: No. My wife is a

5 geneticist,

6   and we sort of are linked to each other in where

7 she

8   goes I go, and where I go she goes. You know,

9 like

10   Ruth and Naomi. So I apologize for that.

11   But the point is that I came to the

12   Children's Hospital of Philadelphia where I was

13   appointed as the chief of nephrology and tasked

14 with

15   the task of creating a dialysis unit and a renal

16   transplant program at that hospital. And I

17 became the

18   chief of the medical staff, and I had

19 appointments

20   in -- as professor of pediatrics, medicine, and

21   urology, and I was also a fellow in the faculty

1 of

2 bi-ethics at the University of Pennsylvania.

3   Q.   And you went to -- just -- I don't

4 know if

5 you put a date on it. Children's Hospital of

6 Philadelphia was in 1987?

7   A.   1987.

8   Q.   And then you retired from there in

9 2016, so

10 if my math is correct, almost 30 years.

11   A.   Yes. Just shy of 30 years.

12   Q.   Okay. And at the time that you

13 authored your

14 two reports in this case -- three reports,

15 excuse me,

16 you were still practicing as a pediatric

17 nephrologist

1   at Children's Hospital of Philadelphia?

2   A.   Correct.

3   Q.   I want to ask you some questions about

4   research that you've conducted on pediatric

5 nephrology

6   issues before you retired.

7   Have you published in the field of

8 pediatric

9   nephrology?

10   A.   I have.

11   Q.   Can you give the special master an

12 idea of

13   the number of publications that you've authored

14 or

15   coauthored.

16   A.   So for some psychological reason, at

17 Penn we

18   were not supposed to number our publications in

19 the CV.

20   I've never figured out why, but they -- if we

21 include

1   chapters, reviews, original peer-reviewed

2   papers,

3   reports, it approaches 400. It's certainly over

4   300.

5   Q.   And getting more specific now, have

6   you

7   authored publications regarding nephrotic

8   syndrome in

9   general?

10   A.   I have.

11   Q.   And any idea, an estimate as to the

12 number of

13   those?

14   A.   It depends on how you want to define

15   nephrotic syndrome, which we shall talk about

16 later.

17   Q.   Okay.

1   A.   But if we're talking about glomerular

2   disorders, somewhere between 40 and 50.

3   Q.   Okay. Have -- as part of your

4   research over

5   the 30-plus -- or almost 30 years or before

6   that, have

7   you been part of any research looking for causes

8   of

9   nephrotic syndrome?

10   A.   Yes. The reason -- one of the main

11   reasons

12   that I went to work in Montreal for Keith

13   Drummond is

14   that Dr. Drummond had worked with Robert Good in

15   Minnesota. And Robert Good was a famous

16   immunologist

17   who actually opened up the whole field of

18   immunopathology. And between Robert Good and

19   Robert

20   Vernier, who was also at the University of

21   Minnesota,

1 they actually laid the basis -- and Marilyn

2 Farquhar

3 of what we now know about renal pathology.

4   And what Dr. Drummond with Dr. Good

5 and

6 others had shown was that in post-streptococcal

7 glomerulonephritis which had been mentioned by

8 Dr. Bellanti yesterday there were immune

9 deposits along

10 the basement membrane -- between the basement

11 membrane

12 and the foot processes. And they also showed

13 that in

14 Goodpasture syndrome, which is a condition that

15 affects

16 the kidneys and the lungs, quite an awful

17 condition,

18 there was an immunological response to the

19 basement

20 membrane of the patient. And the basement

21 membrane was

1   completely replaced by immune deposits.

2   Those that -- were their two -- two of

3   their

4   major achievements at that time. They were

5   unable to

6   show any immune pathology in minimal change

7   nephrotic

8   syndrome. And because they were unable to show

9   any

10   evidence of immune pathology in minimal change

11   nephrology -- nephrotic syndrome, that group in

12   Minnesota and Dr. Drummond's lab started to

13   study the

14   biochemical structure of the basement membrane

15   and to

16   try and understand whether in minimal change

17   nephrotic

18   syndrome, there might be an alteration in the

19   biochemistry of the -- of the basement membrane.

20   Now, of course you can't do that in

21   children,

1   or in adults for that matter. And so they were

2 rat

3   models where we gave the rats an agent called

4   puromycin -- puromycin, p-u-r-o-m-y-c-i-n -- or

5 two

6   anticancer agents. One was daunorubicin, which

7 I can't

8   spell, and another was adriamycin. And the idea

9 was to

10   try and see whether there was structural changes

11 in

12   the -- in isolated glomeruli. And, indeed,

13 there were

14   biochemical changes. And I spent a lot of time

15 doing

16   this work which I did not enjoy at all.

17   What was more interesting was that our

18 group

19   when we saw a little baby with congenital

20 syphilis, we

21   were the first to demonstrate that in this

1 patient's

1   glomeruli, there were immune complexes, that --

2 that

3   these immune complexes contained the antigen

4 derived

5   from the syphilis bacterium. And so we had a

6 direct ·

7   link between the -- the syphilis bacterium and

8 the

9   immune complexes in the kidney.

10   And then a lady was sent to me -- I'm

11 sorry,

12   a young -- a girl about 16 from Newfoundland who

13 had

14   thyroid disease and nephrotic syndrome. And we

15 were

16   able for the first time to show that her immune

17   deposits in her kidney contained thyroid

18 antigen, so we

19   could link these two conditions. And similar

20 study was

21   done on a patient with -- with candida infection

1 who

2   had another form of nephrotic syndrome, and the

3 candida

4   antigen was demonstrated in her -- in the

5 deposits in

6   her kidney.

7   But these patients did not have

8 minimal

9   change nephrotic syndrome. These patients were

10   completely different to minimal change nephrotic

11   syndrome, and the only -- as Dr. Bellanti

12 pointed out

13   yesterday correctly, the only thing they have in

14 common

15   is the fact that they have a lot of protein in

16 the

17   urine and the sequelae of the fact that there is

18 a lot

19   of protein in the urine.

20   Now, I was struck by the fact that we

21 were

1   seeing children with minimal change nephrotic

2 syndrome

1   and that we lived on Sir Lawrence River and all

2 its

3   tributaries in a -- in an area of Canada which -

4 - in

5   which there was a tremendous forestry industry

6 and that

7   there was tremendous contamination by mercury.

8 And

9   there had been reports early on in the '60s that

10 some

11   children with nephrotic syndrome had high levels

12 of

13   mercury. So I looked in our patients to see if

14 I could

15   replicate that, and I was unsuccessful. And

16 actually,

17   subsequently, the link between mercury and

18 nephrotic

19   syndrome has been closed or shown in -- in women

20 in

21   Kenya, black women, who like to use mercury

1 ointment to

2   make themselves look whiter, and that caused

3 nephrotic

4   syndrome. And that is another thing that I was

5   interested in.

6   But what happens in Montreal was that

7 when I

8   was working in the adult hospital, we started

9   collecting adults who had cancer, different

10 kinds of

11   cancer, and nephrotic syndrome. And most of

12 these

13   adults had a different form of nephrotic

14 syndrome,

15   which was a membranous form, some of them had

16 minimal

17   change, and we -- we published several papers on

18 that

19   association.

20   In the mid-'70s, I began to wonder

21 about the

1   relationship between renal vein thrombosis,

2 clots in

3   the -- the kidney, and nephrotic syndrome.   And

4 there

1   were all kinds of theories at that time.   The

2 original

3   case had been a runner called Pollock at

4 Cambridge who

5   dropped down dead as a result of clots and was

6 known to

7   have nephrotic syndrome, and that was 150 years

8 ago.

9   And then a South African doctor, Pollock, a

10   nephrologist, got interested in this and he

11 studied

12   cases.   And he said it was Prednisone which

13 caused the

14   venous thrombosis.   And clearly, that is not

15 true.

16   There is no evidence that Prednisone or -- or

17 thiazides

18   or any of the drugs we use render these patients

19 at

20   risk for renal venous thrombosis, or any

21 thrombi.   And

1   what we -- we learned at the time from reviewing

2   the

3   literature, because we didn't do the original

4   studies,

5   and also from subsequently is that there is this

6   imbalance between coagulant factors and

7   anticoagulant

8   factors that can occur in nephrotic syndrome.

9   But I think this is a good point for

10 me to

11 say that this is extremely uncommon in children.

12   SPECIAL MASTER MILLMAN: What is

13 extremely

14 uncommon?

15   THE WITNESS: Clots in people with

16 nephrotic

17 syndrome.

18   SPECIAL MASTER MILLMAN: I see.

19   THE WITNESS: I'm not saying it

20 doesn't

21 occur, but it is uncommon, unlike adults where

1 it

1   occurs more frequently. In fact, one paper in

2   the '70s

3   looked -- one group looked at this very

4   carefully and

5   came to the conclusion that 30 percent of adults

6   with

7   nephrotic syndrome might have a thrombus

8   somewhere in

9   their body, which is tremendously high. And the

10 three

11 that there is such a difference between children

12 and

13 adults is that children with nephrotic syndrome

14 usually

15 do not have proteinuria for a long time. They

16 have a

17 episode and, generally speaking, within two

18 weeks, they

19 respond to treatment and the proteinuria is

20 gone. And

21 so they are not really at risk for developing

1 these

2   clots, and that's why it's so rare.

3   Whereas adults with membranous

4 nephrotic

5   syndrome may have nephrotic syndrome for months

6 or

7   years because there still isn't a good treatment

8 for

9   that, and so they're losing the important

10 things. So

11   the -- the -- there are these coagulants and

12   anticoagulants that are lost and the balance is

13 lost.

14   These patients also have high hemoglobins from

15   steroids, and they have platelets that are high

16 in

17   number and very active. And the whole stage is

18 set for

19   clots, and yet we don't see that very often.

20   And what is even more intriguing is

21 that both

1   in the adult literature, but especially in the

2   pediatric literature, one hardly ever sees

3 arterial

1   clots as occurred in JM. In fact, in the

2   pediatric literature, the ratio of -- of -- of

3 venous

4   to arterial clots is 20 to 1. In adults, it's

5 about 3

6   to 1. And of course there are reasons why

7 adults might

8   have clots, because of arthrosclerosis, smoking,

9   obesity, all of those other factors. Anyhow,

10 that was

11   my interest in the coagulation abnormalities in

12   nephrotic syndrome.

13   And then I started to become

14 profoundly

15   interested in the genetic basis of the nephrotic

16   syndrome. And my -- my interest was piqued

17 because we

18   had a number of families where the mother and

19 the child

20   had nephrotic syndrome or two children had

21 nephrotic

1   syndrome, and these were cases of minimal change

2   nephrotic syndrome. There were other cases in

3 which

4   there was focal sclerosis. And I was very

5 fortunate to

6   be able to collaborate with people at Harvard,

7 and we

8   were able to show in some of our patients that

9 patients

10   with focal sclerosis have a mutation in a gene

11 for

12   podocin, a gene for podocin and for alpha 4 --

13 I'm

14   sorry, alpha-actinin 4.

15   Now, Dr. Bellanti, with great respect,

16 made a

17   misstatement yesterday which I would like to

18 correct on

19   the record. He said that the genetic causes of

20   nephrotic syndrome occur in neonates and infants

21 and

1   not in older people. This is a very old idea

2 which is

3   now being completely shown to be wrong. He is

4 quite

5   correct that there are a number of inherited

6 conditions

7   in which babies are born with nephrotic

8 syndrome, and

9   there are mutations for a gene called nephrin

10 and

11   others, and there are syndromes where there are

12 babies

13   with nephrotic syndrome. And we, indeed, have

14   described some of those conditions and helped

15   to -- well, sent people -- DNA to help define

16 the

17   genetic basis of those conditions.

18   But what is much more important is

19 that we

20   have families and everybody now knows that a

21 large

1   number -- well, 30 percent of the patients with

2 focal

3   sclerosis of whatever age, but not babies or

4 infants,

5   older children, adults will have mutations. And

6 there

7   are more than 20 mutations that have been found

8 so far.

9   And these mutations are in proteins that help to

10   control the -- the podocyte that Dr. Bellanti

11 showed us

12   yesterday, which is an extraordinary cell that

13 sits on

14   the outer surface of the basement membrane and

15 which

16   controls the basement membrane. You can see it

17 in

18   video recordings, and -- and monitors the

19 basement

20   membrane, improves its structure, contributes to

21 its

1   function.

2   And it has these interdigitating

3 processes

1   which are set up in such a way that they're like

2 rafts

3   of nephrin and podocin, and they are of a

4 certain

5   caliber, a caliber which impedes the passage of

6   albumin. And if there is a disruption in this -

7 - this

8   apparatus, albumin can pass through and

9 nephrotic

10   syndrome can occur. And of course, in minimal

11 change

12   nephrotic syndrome, it is predominantly albumin

13 that is

14   lost, because the damage to the -- the kidney in

15   minimal change nephrotic syndrome is so

16 minuscule in

17   the sense of being demonstrative -- demonstrated

18 by

19   light microscopy, by electron microscopy, that

20 albumin

21   only gets through, mainly albumin. In the

1 membranous

2   form of nephrotic syndrome and the other forms

3 where

4   there are immune complexes that disrupt the --

5 the

6   architecture of the foot processes, there's

7 massive

8   leakage of all kinds of protein not just

9 albumin.

10   So we -- we were quite excited about

11 all

12   that. And we also were able to show in a

13 publication

14   about two years ago, I think, that it turned out

15 to be

16   a little girl who -- whose father is a

17 pediatrician --

18   grandfather's a pediatrician. And for some

19 reason, he

20   didn't feel comfortable about her, and he found

21 that

1   she had leukemia.   And she was treated, and she

2   relapsed, and she was put onto one of these

3 magical new

4   drugs called tyrosine kinase inhibitor and she

5 went

1   into remission. And then she was sent to me

2 because

3   she had nephrotic syndrome.

4   And I had a tremendous argument with

5 the

6   oncologist, not the first I've lost, where I

7 said she

8   had minimal change nephrotic syndrome. We

9 should treat

10   her with Prednisone. And they said, Oh, no.

11 She might

12   have a side effect of the tyrosine kinase

13 inhibitor.

14   To prove my point, I biopsied her, because I

15 thought

16   she would have horrible disease, and she had

17 minimal

18   changes, no changes.

19   And although I was afraid when they

20 stopped

21   the tyrosine kinase inhibitor that her leukemia

1 would

2   relapse, in fact the nephrotic syndrome went

3 away and

4   her leukemia relapsed and she had a bone marrow

5   transplant. And we had one or two other such

6 cases,

7   and there have been reports of that in the adult

8   literature. An example of how you can see what

9 looks

10   like minimal change nephrotic syndrome that has

11 nothing

12   to do with immune complexes or abnormalities in

13 the

14   immune system. And I will come back to that

15 later.

16   So I don't want to take up too much

17 time and

18   tell you about all the other studies we did on -

19 - on

20   genetic metabolic disorders where we defined

21 some of

1   the glomerular changes.   I don't want to go to

2 that,

3   but just to mention that.

1   But there is one very fascinating

2 observation

3   which we made which is our own original

4 observation

5   where there's a genetic condition called Dent

6 disease

7   which is called a channelopathy. And these

8 patients

9   have what's called Fanconi syndrome, and they

10 get

11   kidney stones and they go into kidney failure.

12 And we

13   biopsied them and noticed that they had focal

14   sclerosis. And what we've seen now is that you

15 can

16   have these metabolic disorders where the end

17 result is

18   focal sclerosis, not just Dent disease but other

19   metabolic disorders as well.

20   So that, in a nutshell, is I think

21 what I

1   want to say about my research and publications.

2   Q.   Just a few additional questions.

3   In your practice when -- before you

4 retired

5   in 2016, it sounds obvious that you treated

6 patients

7   with -- children with nephrotic syndrome?

8   A.   I remember the first child I saw with

9   nephrotic syndrome in 1966. I remember her so

10 well

11 because she was treated with Prednisone.

12   And, Special Master, we physicians do

13 terrible things. We didn't have a clue how to

14 use

15 Prednisone. And this poor little thing was

16 stunted,

17 dwarfed.

18   SPECIAL MASTER MILLMAN: And fat.

1   THE WITNESS: Fat, with marks on her

2 face.

3   Quite awful. And one of the reasons why

4 families have

5   allergies, are allergic to Prednisone and why I

6 love

7   Prednisone, but hate it, because of the side

8 effects.

9   And that was my -- she was my first patient as

10 an

11   intern. And in those barbaric days, we used to

12 drain

13   the peritoneal fluid that she had accumulated

14 and

15   infuse it into her to try to get her stable. It

16 was

17   quite primitive.

18   But since then, in Johannesburg in a

19 white

20   hospital and a black hospital, in Montreal in

21 Great

1   Hall Street in London where I worked as a

2 visiting

3   professor, and in Philadelphia, I have been

4 involved in

5   the care of hundreds and hundreds and hundreds

6 of

7   children with nephrotic syndrome, including many

8   hundreds of children with minimal change or

9 steroid

10   sensitive nephrotic syndrome.

11   BY MR. WISHARD:

12   Q.   We'll talk about that.

13   A.   And thousands and thousands of

14 relapses.

15   Q.   And you've testified several times

16 before on

17   the vaccine program I believe; correct?

18   A.   I have, yes. Twice.

19   Q.   And outside of the vaccine program,

20 have you

21   worked as an expert?

1   A.   I do some work as an expert, but at

2 the

3   moment, I have, I think, three ongoing cases,

4 about

5   three to four cases a year.

6   Q.   Some for plaintiffs, some for

7 defendants?

8   A.   It's the defendants that seek me out

9 for some

10   reason. But I do do plaintiff work as well,

11 yes. And

12   I was able to help a little girl with nephrotic

13   syndrome's family get her considerable award a

14 few

15   years ago, yes.

16   MR. WISHARD: I would offer Dr. Kaplan

17 as an

18   expert in pediatric nephrology subject to any

19   cross-examination.

20   SPECIAL MASTER MILLMAN: Mr. McHugh?

21   MR. McHUGH: No objection.

1   SPECIAL MASTER MILLMAN: Okay.

2 Remember if

3   you're going to talk from the end of the

4 courtroom, you

5   need a microphone.

6   MR. McHUGH: No objection.

7   SPECIAL MASTER MILLMAN: Thank you.

8   He's so admitted.

9   MR. WISHARD: Thank you.

10   BY MR. WISHARD:

11   Q.   Dr. Kaplan, you were asked a while

12 ago, and

13   you were being asked again today, to review this

14 case

15   and give your opinions.

1   And have you had a chance to review

2 all of

3   the exhibits that have been filed by the parties

4 in

5   this case, medical records, expert reports, and

6 the

7   medical literature?

8   A.   Yes, sir.

9   Q.   And obviously you were here yesterday.

10 You

11   heard all the testimony that was presented,

12 including

13   the PowerPoint presentation that was done by

14   Dr. Bellanti?

15   A.   Yes, sir.

16   Q.   And have you reached opinions on the

17 claim

18   that petitioners have made that the flu vaccine

19   significantly aggravated JM's nephrotic

20 syndrome,

21   and specifically minimal change disease? Have

1 you

2 reached opinions?

3   A.   I have, sir.

4   Q.   And I know some of those opinions are

5 set

6 forth in your reports which are Exhibits A, G,

7 and L,

8 but I'm not really going to get into those

9 today.   I'm

10 going to talk beyond the reports.

11   But have you -- I'm going to ask you

12 several

13 opinions up front, and then I want to talk a

14 little bit

15 about some general things and go into the

16 opinions in

17 specific.

18   Based on your review of the evidence,

19 in your

1   view, to a more likely than not standard, did

2   the

3   October 1, 2009, flu vaccine significantly

4   aggravate

5   JM's nephrotic syndrome or minimal change

6   disease?

7   A.   No, sir.

8   Q.   In your opinion, did the October 1,

9   2009, flu

10   vaccination in any way aggravate his nephrotic

11   syndrome

12   minimal change disease to then cause, 22 months

13   later,

14   the CVA that he had?

15   A.   Absolutely not.

16   Q.   There are lots of terms used yesterday

17   from a

18   nephrotic standpoint, and I think I want to go

19   through

20   just a couple of those with you just to make

21   sure that

1   we have the definitions down. And you talked

2   about

3   what nephrotic syndrome is, and I think you

4   talked

5   earlier about -- you talked about your research

6   of what

7   minimal change disease is.

8   But do you have anything to add to

9   that in

10   terms of definition from your viewpoint of

11   nephrotic

12   syndrome and minimal change disease?

13   A.   Thank you. Well, Special Master asked

14   about

15   the terms steroid sensitive and steroid

16   resistant

17   nephrotic syndrome and steroid dependent

18   nephrotic

19   syndrome. And I would like to amplify or talk

20   more

21   about Dr. Quan's explanation, and I have no

1   disagreement with Dr. Quan's explanation.

1   When I started looking after patients

2 with

3   nephrotic syndrome, it was the custom to biopsy

4 them.

5   A nephrologist was almost like a carpenter with

6 a

7   hammer. Every time we saw a kidney, we biopsied

8 it.

9   And it became apparent that this wasn't the

10 right thing

11   to do, that maybe we should give each patient --

12 and

13   we're talking about pediatrics now, because the

14 --

15   the -- the percentages of different types of

16 nephrotic

17   syndrome are different in children versus

18 adults. We

19   should give them a trial of steroids for up to

20 six

21   weeks and see if they respond. And if they

1 respond, we

2   would call them steroid sensitive. And if they

3 didn't

4   within that six-week period, we'd call them

5 steroid

6   resistant.

7   And of course, this just didn't

8 happen. It

9   was based on a lot of thinking by people. And

10 it

11   became apparent that the majority, but not all,

12 the

13   patients who were steroid sensitive had minimal

14 change

15   nephrotic syndrome. And that the majority of

16 the

17   patients who were steroid resistant had focal

18   sclerosis. Because clinically, it's virtually

19   impossible to differentiate between the two.

20 You can

21   really only do it with a kidney biopsy or the

1 response

2   to steroids, and it's really important to know.

3 So

4   patients with membranous glomerulopathy or focal

1   sclerosis or membranoproliferative

2 glomerulonephritis,

3   other kinds of nephrotic syndrome do not respond

4 to

5   Prednisone or respond poorly to Prednisone and

6 they're

7   resistant.

8   It became apparent that although the

9 majority

10   of patients with steroid with what was minimal

11 change

12   nephrotic syndrome, would respond within a

13 reasonable

14   time, usually within two to three weeks, to

15 steroids if

16   given in the right dose. Some of them could not

17 be

18   weaned off the steroids. And what they would do

19 is

20   they -- what they do is they -- they have what

21 we call

1   blips or breakthroughs where the parents are

2 measuring

3   the urine, checking the urine protein every day,

4 find

5   there's proteinuria for a day or two or three,

6 and then

7   the child improves or not. You sometimes have

8 to

9   increase the dose of the Prednisone. And those

10   steroid-dependent patients may be very, very

11 difficult

12   to get off steroids. And the exact reasons are

13 not

14   well understood.

15   But then there are patients who are

16   exquisitely sensitive to Prednisone. They do

17 what

18   they're supposed to do and they go into

19 remission. And

20   then subsequently later, a year later, several

21 years

1   later, for inexplicable reasons, they become

2 steroid

3   resistant or steroid dependent.   And those are

4 the

1   patients where we decide to biopsy them as did

2 Dr. Quan

3   in JM's case. Because we would worry that they

4   don't have typical minimal change nephrotic

5 syndrome,

6   but they may have focal sclerosis. And he even

7   included IGA nephropathy as a possibility.

8   And we then have to take another step,

9 which

10 is to decide which additional agent to put the

11 patient

12 on. And we have used high dosage intravenous

13 steroids

14 to get them into remission. We've done that

15 successfully, the protocols for that. We have -

16 - we

17 have given them Cytoxan, which we don't use

18 anymore

19 because it has horrible side effects. And we

20 have used

21 Prograf. I'll use the term Prograf for the rest

1 of

2   this discussion.

3   And Prograf, unfortunately, can -- if

4 used

5   in -- in a dose that's too high or for a very

6 long

7   time, it can cause damage to the kidney, to the

8 tubules

9   of the kidney. But actually, it can even cause

10 damage

11 that looks like focal sclerosis. Despite that,

12 patients who have had liver transplants or

13 kidney

14 transplants may be placed on Prograf for life.

15 And

16 people accept that there may be some damage to

17 the

18   kidney.

19   So once they've been on Prograf, they

20 may

21 become dependent on Prograf. Or in some cases,

1 when

1   they're weaned off the Prograf, they may become

2 steroid

3   sensitive again. Or they may remain in

4 remission for

5   prolonged periods of time. And that's why I

6 have used

7   the term that minimal change nephrotic syndrome

8 behaves

9   in a chaotic way.

10   I had a patient once, Ms. Green, who

11 had

12   nephrotic syndrome. I treated her and I never

13 saw her

14   again. And being very sensitive about things, I

15   thought they had gone to the opposition. And

16 one

17   day --

18   SPECIAL MASTER MILLMAN: You mean

19 another

20   doctor?

21   THE WITNESS: Huh?

1   SPECIAL MASTER MILLMAN: You mean

2 another

3   doctor?

4   THE WITNESS: Another hospital, yeah.

5   And ten years later, I was in a

6 delicatessen,

7   and I heard this woman yelling at me, Dr.

8 Kaplan,

9   Dr. Kaplan. She told me who she was. She said

10 she's

11   the mother of this child that's ten years and

12 the

13   child's never had a relapse. And two weeks

14 later, she

15   called me and she said, I wish I hadn't seen

16 you.

17   She's just relapsed for the first time.

18   So it is unpredictable. It's chaotic.

19 But

20   in an attempt to try and undue the chaos, some

21 people

1   have tried to find predictive factors which

2 you'll ask

3   me about later to remind me.

4   Now, steroid resistant nephrotic

5 syndrome in

6   this context is usually associated with focal

7 segmental

8   glomerulosclerosis.

9   Q.   FSGS.

10   A.   FSGS.

11   Q.   Okay.

12   A.   And, again, with great respect, I want

13 to

14   correct Dr. Bellanti for something he said

15 yesterday.

16   I just want to set the record straight. He said

17 that

18   when he was much younger than he and I both are

19 at this

20   time, he had encountered patients with diabetes

21 who had

1   nodular sclerosis in their kidneys.   That is a

2   completely different condition.   Completely

3 different

4   pathophysiology to focal segmental

5 glomerulosclerosis.

6   Focal segmental glomerulosclerosis is

7 not

8   minimal change nephrotic syndrome.   It is focal

9   segmental glomerulosclerosis.   It has mutations

10 that

11   have not been found in minimal change nephrotic

12   syndrome.   It has a course which is almost

13 always --

14   always ends in kidney transplant, and it is not

15 minimal

16   change nephrotic syndrome.

17   SPECIAL MASTER MILLMAN: Why is the

18 disease

19   minimal change nephrotic syndrome called minimal

1   change?

2   THE WITNESS: Initially, it was called

3 Nil

4   disease.

5   SPECIAL MASTER MILLMAN: It was called

6 what?

7   THE WITNESS: Nil, N-i-l.

8   SPECIAL MASTER MILLMAN: Nil, like

9 nothing?

10   THE WITNESS: Yes.

11   SPECIAL MASTER MILLMAN: Nothing

12 disease?

13   THE WITNESS: Nothing.

14   And the reason -- well, you know --

15 you know,

16   physicians are very cute. They -- they -- they

17 talk

18   about strawberry tongues and bread and butter

19 hearts,

20   and they use all kinds of terminology which we

21 try not

1   to use anymore. So somebody was being cute and

2 called

3   it Nil disease. And the reason it was called

4 Nil

5   disease or minimal change is that if you were to

6 put

7   two microscopes side by side, a biopsy from a

8 child

9   with nephrotic syndrome, with minimal change

10 disease,

11   and a normal child's, somebody who has died, for

12   example, in the other microscope, you would see

13 no

14   change, no difference on --

15   SPECIAL MASTER MILLMAN: They look the

16 same?

17   THE WITNESS: Absolutely the same on

18 light

19   microscope. When you look at it with a light

20   microscope and you do special stains, you see

1   absolutely no difference. And specifically,

2 Special

3   Master, you do not see any increase in the

4 number of

5   cells in the kidney, in the glomerulus, none of

6 the --

7   the immunologically active cells, the T cells,

8 the

9   B cells, the Th, whatever cells are increased in

10 the

11   patients with minimal change nephrotic syndrome.

12 You

13   don't see them. And you don't see necrosis or

14 death of

15   any tissue which you see in other kinds of

16 nephritis.

17   You don't see fibrin deposits. You -- all you

18 see in

19   the light microscopic view is a normal

20 glomerulus.

21   So then people start -- for example,

1 my

2   mentor, Dr. Drummond and his group, they stained

3 these

4   glomeruli for hemoglobins, IGG, IGA, IGM and of

5 course

6   complement. And none of that was present in the

7   children with classical minimal change nephrotic

8   syndrome.

9   And when these biopsies were examined

10 under

11   the ultra -- the electron microscope, they found

12 that

13   the foot processes of the podocytes instead of

14 being

15   discretely separate from each other had become

16 effaced.

17   SPECIAL MASTER MILLMAN: Effaced

18 meaning?

19   THE WITNESS: E-f-f-a-c-e-d.

20   SPECIAL MASTER MILLMAN: Meaning what?

21   THE WITNESS: At first, the term they

1 used

2   was fused, because it looked as though they had

3 just

 1   become one cell or one component of the cell.

 2 But

 3   actually, there are studies that show that this

 4 is a

 5   very dynamic process and reversible. So what

 6 that led

 7   to was the notion that between these foot

 8 processes,

 9   something was keeping these foot processes or

10 these

11   interdigitations apart and that that changed.

12   And one of the things we studied and

13 other

14   people studied was the fact that these foot

15 processes

16   were embedded in something called sialoprotein,

17   s-i-a-l-o-p-r-o-t-e-i-n, which is negatively

18 charged.

19   It's the sialoprotein which coats platelets and

20 red

21   cells and other cells that prevents them from

1 adhering

2   or sticking to each other. And interestingly

3 enough,

4   albumin is also negatively charged. So when we

5 talk

6   about the impedance to the passage of albumin

7 through

8   the kidney, we are talking about the size of the

9 foot

10   process pores, but also the charge.

11   Now, the thing is, what I didn't

12 understand

13   was if these foot processes became fused or

14 effaced,

15   how could the albumin get through? But actually

16 what

17   happens is that the foot processes became

18 effaced and

19   they lifted off the basement membrane. And so

20 whereas

21   before you had a cell which was monitoring the

1   trafficking through that membrane, there were

2 parts of

3   that membrane were now demuted and there was no

1   podocyte to monitor it and protein would pass

2   through.

3   And there are very elegant studies that show how

4   this

5   has been shown to be the case.

6   SPECIAL MASTER MILLMAN: Does

7   glomeruli mean

8   kidney cell or something else?

9   THE WITNESS: So each kidney has

10 around

11 1 million nephrons. And the nephron consists of

12 a

13 glomerulus, which is a little round structure.

14 It's a

15 network of capillaries. It has what's known as

16 an

17 afferent arterial through which the blood goes

18 to this

19 network and an efferent arterial which takes the

20 blood

21 back to the circulation. And in this

1 glomerulus, in

2   these capillaries in the glomerulus, of which

3 there are

4   a million of these, this glomerulus is able to

5 keep red

6   cells, white cells, albumin, proteins in the

7   bloodstream and allow water to filter, not only

8 water,

9   but all the chemicals we want to get rid of.

10 Like

11   urea, creatinine, potassium, whatever we need to

12 get

13   rid of.

14   And that -- those chemicals will be

15 filtered.

16   They'll go into this extraordinary structure

17 called the

18   tubule where all kinds of things are happening,

19   absorption, reabsorption, excretion, a balancing

20 of the

21   body's fluid. And, in fact, in an adult, 180

1 liters of

2 water get filtered by the kidneys each day.

3 180, and

1   yet the kidney is able to -- to put into the

2 toilet

3   between 1 and 2 liters of water a day. So 98

4 percent

5   of all the fluid that's filtered is reabsorbed.

6 That's

7   actually quite an amazing structure.

8   SPECIAL MASTER MILLMAN: Is the

9 minimal

10   change in the minimal change nephrotic syndrome

11 the

12   leaking through of the albumin only and that's

13 the

14   protein count?

15   THE WITNESS: So you have -- you have

16 a habit

17   of asking interesting questions.

18   The -- under normal circumstances, we

19 all

20   leak protein into our urine. In fact, we leak

21 albumin

1   into our urine. Normal people do, but small

2   quantities. In minimal change nephrotic

3 syndrome, the

4   predominantly protein that leaks into the urine

5 is the

6   albumin.

7   But interestingly enough, it leaks IGG

8 and

9   IGA I think, because in nephrotics, the IGG

10 levels can

11   be really quite low. The IGA levels can be

12 quite low

13   because of the loss of these proteins in the

14 urine.

15   And also, of course, all the other proteins,

16 like the

17   proteins that carry thyroid hormone and other

18 hormones,

19   and I don't want to go on. But yes, mainly

20 albumin in

21   minimal change nephrotic syndrome.

1   SPECIAL MASTER MILLMAN: Okay.   I

2 don't know

1   where you were, but proceed.

2   THE WITNESS: I'm sorry.

3   SPECIAL MASTER MILLMAN: No, no,

4   that's okay.

5   BY MR. WISHARD:

6   Q.   Just wanted to finish up.

7   Are there any other terms or

8   definitions that

9   you would want to clear up or talk about before

10 we move

11 on or talk about JM's case?

12   A.   I do want to come back to membranous

13 nephrotic syndrome.

14   Q.   Okay.

15   A.   Mainly because of the respondent's

16 production

17 of a few reports.

18   Q.   Respondent is us. You mean --

19   A.   I mean petitioners. I wrote it down,

20 and I

21 got it wrong. The petitioner's --

1   SPECIAL MASTER MILLMAN: That's all

2   right.

3   That's okay.   We're all here to help each other.

4   THE WITNESS: The petitioner's

5   production of

6   a few case reports in which there were a few

7   adults who

8   developed nephrotic syndrome and allegedly as a

9   result

10   of receiving a flu vaccine.   And in those cases,

11 as one

12   would expect in an adult population, there were

13 only a

14   few cases, but they were mainly focal sclerosis

15 and

16   membranous.

1   BY MR. WISHARD:

2   Q.   When you say focal sclerosis, are you

3   referring to FSGS?

4   A.   I'm sorry, FSGS.

5   Q.   That's fine, FSGS, which JM does not

6   have.

7   A.   No.   And the reason why I want to come

8 back

9   to membranous is because the most common

10 acquired cause

11   of membranous nephrotic syndrome in the world is

12 a

13   viral infection called hepatitis B.   And

14 hepatitis B is

15   an accepted, well-defined cause of membranous

16   nephropathy.   And there you have the virus, you

17 have

18   the antigen of the virus demonstrated in the

19 immune

20   complexes, and that particular well-documented

21   viral-induced kidney disease is not minimal

1 change.

2 And the same is true for hepatitis C which

3 causes

4 another kind of -- of -- of glomeruli disorder,

5 but not

6 minimal change. And I just wanted to make that

7 point

8 clearly.

9   Q.   You also, I think, wanted to explain

10 the

11 difference, correct, on nephritic which is a

12 term that

13 came up yesterday versus nephrotic.

14   A.   Yes. So the nephrotic syndrome is

15 defined as

16 has been defined by Dr. Quan, and Dr. Bellanti

17 repeated

18 this, by the fact the predominance abnormality

19 is the

1   albumin in the urine. And the people with

2 nephritis or

3   nephritic syndrome, they have blood in the urine

4 as

5   well. There's protein in the urine.

6   SPECIAL MASTER MILLMAN: Because

7 that's an

8   inflammatory disease?

9   THE WITNESS: It's an inflammatory

10 disease.

11   It is a -- it is a group of inflammatory

12 diseases,

13   post-streptococcal glomerulonephritis being one

14 of them

15   in which there is infiltration into the kidney

16 of

17   leukocytes and other immunoreactive cells.

18 They're

19   immune deposits and they have blood in the

20 urine.

21   Interestingly enough, there is an

1 inherited

2 condition which may be indistinguishable from

3 glomerulonephritis called Alport syndrome.

4   SPECIAL MASTER MILLMAN: Who?

5   THE WITNESS: Alport, A-l-p-o-r-t.

6 Alport

7 syndrome. It's called hereditary nephritis with

8 deafness described by a South African many years

9 ago.

10 And Alport syndrome is the result of a

11 biochemical

12 structural change in the basement membrane. Not

13 in the

14 foot processes, not in the podocyte primarily,

15 but in

16 the basement membrane itself.

17   And people with Alport syndrome have

18 proteinuria. And they can have nephrotic

19 syndrome.

20 And the way we treat them is we put them onto

21 Vasotec,

1   which is an ACE inhibitor. And I want to come

2 back and

3   talk about Vasotec later if you remind me

4 because it's

5   very important.

6   We also treat them -- we can treat

7 them

8   with -- with cyclosporine or Prograf which are

9   so-called immunosuppressant agents which help to

10 reduce

11   the protein in the urine in this condition with

12 a

13   structural abnormality where nobody has ever

14 hinted

15   that there's an immunological basis for that

16 particular

17   condition.

18   SPECIAL MASTER MILLMAN: Are you

19 saying that

20   except for Alports --

21   THE WITNESS: Yes.

1   SPECIAL MASTER MILLMAN: -- condition,

2   minimal change nephrotic syndrome is not an

3   inflammatory disease?

4   THE WITNESS: There is absolutely no

5 evidence

6   that it's inflammatory, ma'am, and there is --

7 there

8   is -- there is -- speaking as a pseudo

9 immunologist not

10   a real immunologist, if you look at the --

11 whatever you

12   would look for, you don't see any changes. The

13   complement is not decreased. The immunoglobulin

14 levels

15   are actually decreased. There are no

16 circulating

17   immune complexes. There are no infiltrates of

18 cells

19   into the glomerulus to make it an inflammatory

1   condition. There are no immune complexes in the

2   kidney. It is not an inflammatory condition,

3 ma'am.

4   SPECIAL MASTER MILLMAN: Would you

5 define

6   complement which, just to remind the court

7 reporter, is

8   c-o-m-p-l-e-m-e-n-t.

9   THE WITNESS: Yeah. Complements is a

10 -- a

11   cascade of proteins and enzymes. On the one

12 hand,

13   there is the complement pathway. It's called

14 the

15   classical complement pathway. Classical. And

16 on the

17   other side there is the alternate pathway. Just

18 as

19   with coagulation, there is -- there are checks

20 and

21   balances. And in the complement system, what

1 the

2   complement does, it helps to opsonize bacteria.

3 It

4   helps to make a sandwich of the bacteria with

5   immunoglobulins and punch holes into the wall of

6 the

7   bacteria and destroy them.

8   And in the kidney, what happens in the

9 kidney

10   in those conditions in which complement is

11 present,

12   such as membranous GN or streptococcal

13   glomerulonephritis, there is activation of

14 complements

15   to form what is known as the membrane attack

16 complex

17   which is what it is. It's a complex of about

18 five

19   different complements, proteins, which kill

20 bacteria or

21   they punch holes in -- in cells or in membranes.

1   SPECIAL MASTER MILLMAN: If someone, a

2 child

429

1   let's say, has minimal change disease and the

2 child

3   gets a virus, maybe a flu virus, maybe something

4 else,

5   does his minimal change disease get worse?

6   THE WITNESS: In what sense, ma'am?

7   SPECIAL MASTER MILLMAN: Well, does it

8 worsen

9   the disease because now he's sick with the flu

10 virus?

11   THE WITNESS: Well, the flu virus is

12 going to

13   make him pretty sick. There's no question about

14 that.

15   Does -- does it have a different outcome? I

16 don't

17   think so. I -- I -- I have not seen that. And

18 I have

19   not read of any -- read anything that anybody

20 has ever

21   said that the flu virus in any way changes the

1 course

2 of the nephrotic syndrome or the severity of the

3 nephrotic syndrome.

4   SPECIAL MASTER MILLMAN: So if JM's

5 nephrologist, first Dr. Seikaly, Dr. Quan,

6 recommend

7 that he get flu vaccines so he wouldn't actually

8 get

9 the flu virus, it wasn't because they were

10 concerned

11 about it having -- if he were sick, having an

12 effect on

13 his minimal change disease?

14   THE WITNESS: This -- this gets us

15 into quite

16 a complicated subject. As Dr. Quan said, most

17 pediatric nephrologists have this heard memory

18 or idea

19 that relapses may be triggered by a flu -- a

20 virus

21 infection like a flu virus.

1   And so as a pediatric nephrologist, I

2 would

3   say to mothers, We should vaccinate your child.

4 Who --

5   who wants your child -- do you really want your

6 child

7   to get sick with flu? And most of the mothers

8 would

9   say, Absolutely not. So I can't give you a

10 figure, but

11   large numbers of the patients were not

12 vaccinated

13   against the flu virus, and I went along with

14 that

15   because you learn not to argue with mothers.

16 You --

17   what you do say to them is, You don't want your

18 child

19   to get chickenpox because that's a different

20 story or

21   measles or polio, tetanus. So let's bargain.

1 Let's go

2   with those immunizations. The flu virus, well,

3 your

4   child might get very, very sick from the flu.

5 It's not

6   going to do anything to the nephrotic syndrome.

7   So when I'm asked, and I bring this up

8 now

9   because you raised the point, do I think that

10 the --

11   the vaccine in any way changed JM's course, I

12   would have to say looking at his case, I don't

13 think

14   so. But thinking about my patients, I don't

15 really

16   know which of my patients who had relapses were

17   relapsing having had the flu vaccine or not. I

18 just

19   don't know.

20   What I do know, ma'am, is that in the

21 entire

1   literature, there is not a single case report,

2 not even

3   a case report, of a child developing minimal

4 change

1   nephrotic syndrome following the flu vaccine or

2   relapsing following the flu vaccine.

3   Now, you might think, well, maybe

4   there's

5   some reason we don't study this. But why

6   wouldn't we

7   if it were an important thing? And in addition

8   to

9   that, ma'am, in the past 20 years, and I have

10 gone to

11 the CDC records to look at this, either 2

12 billion or

13 more than 2 billion flu vaccines have been given

14 in the

15 United States alone. And the incidence of

16 minimal

17 change nephrotic syndrome has remained

18 absolutely

19 stable. In fact, there are a few studies in

20 adults

21 which show that focal sclerosis has increased,

1 and

2   that's for other reasons, but minimal change in

3 adults

4   has remained absolutely stable. So I can't see

5 the

6   link. Are they epidemiologically, and with due

7   respect, immunologically between the flu virus

8 and

9   onset of nephrotic syndrome or relapse -- I'm

10 sorry the

11   vaccine, between the vaccine with onset or

12 relapse, and

13   I do not believe that nephrotic syndrome is part

14 and

15   parcel of the disease called influenza.

16   If -- if you said to me, What is

17 influenza?

18   Is pneumonia part of influenza? I would say,

19 Oh, yeah.

20   Is meningitis and cephalitis part of influenza?

21 I

1   would say, Absolutely. But is nephrotic

2 syndrome part

3   of it? Not at all.

1   SPECIAL MASTER MILLMAN: Because of

2 this

3   program, we see lots and lots of -- of illnesses

4 come

5   before the special masters.

6   THE WITNESS: Yes.

7   SPECIAL MASTER MILLMAN: So I'm used

8 to

9   thinking in terms of an inflammatory disease.

10   Sometimes we call things immune mediated.

11 Sometimes we

12   call them autoimmune. Sometimes it's just an

13   inflammatory disease. It could be

14 rheumatological. It

15   could be neurological. I'm sure I'm leaving out

16 a

17   whole world of things out there. But you just

18 said

19   earlier, I think, in your direct testimony that

20 in

21   children minimal change nephrotic syndrome, it's

1 not an

2 inflammatory disease.

3   Is it also not an immune-mediated

4 disease?

5   THE WITNESS: If you walked into this

6 room

7 yesterday from another galaxy where two neutrons

8 --

9 what are they called, kilo plata something.

10   SPECIAL MASTER MILLMAN: Kilonova.

11   THE WITNESS: Kilonova collided, and

12 Einstein

13 predicted that if you set up the LIGO system,

14 there

15 would be waves that come through the universe,

16 and one

17 day we would pick up the fact that these --

18   SPECIAL MASTER MILLMAN: We have gold,

19 silver, and uranium thanks to this.

1   THE WITNESS: Right. I would love to

2   understand that.

3   But you said that once upon a time,

4 people

5   talked about immunological basis of minimal

6 change

7   nephrotic syndrome as I myself did. But the

8 world has

9   changed. And it's changed very dramatically.

10 And we

11   have to take into consideration those changes

12 that have

13   occurred. And those changes relate to our whole

14 new

15   understanding of the biology of the podocytes,

16 what

17   it -- what its structure is, its sarcoskeleton,

18 what

19   maintains it, how it functions in terms of

20 preventing

21   proteinuria, and all the genes that are

1 involved.

2   And the fact that although people

3 still say

4   that Prednisone acts as an immunosuppressant in

5   nephrotic syndrome or that Prograf acts as an

6   immunosuppressant in nephrotic syndrome,

7 firstly, there

8   is absolutely no evidence for that whatsoever.

9 And

10   secondly, there is increasing evidence that

11 Prednisone

12   acts through angiopoietin 4, a-n-g-i-o-p-o-i-e-

13 t-i-n 4,

14   which is a chemical compound in the basement

15 membrane,

16   and that cyclosporin acts by stabilizing the

17 podocytes,

18   and that there are so many other receptors and -

19 - and

20   proteins that are affected by different agents

21 that

1   people thought were immunologically mediated but

2 more

3   and more seem not to be immunologically

4 mediated.

1   And if I may digress just a little

2 bit,

3 because I wanted to make this point as clearly

4 as I

5 can. There is an agent called Vasotec. It's

6 also -- a

7 cousin of Vasotec is enalapril.

8   SPECIAL MASTER MILLMAN: Is this a

9 drug?

10   THE WITNESS: Yes, ma'am.

11   SPECIAL MASTER MILLMAN: Okay.

12   THE WITNESS: These are drugs that are

13 used

14 to treat high blood pressure, hypertension. The

15 one is

16 an ACE inhibitor. It inhibits an enzyme that's

17 important in raising peptides that cause high

18 blood

19 pressure, and the other blocks the action of

20 these

21 peptides. And there's no question that these

1 blood

2   pressure medications lower blood pressure and

3 became

4   very popular in nephrology. And people noticed

5 in

6   diabetics, focal sclerosis, patients Alport

7 syndrome

8   that if you use these agents, here are the two

9 thoughts

10   to be antihypertensive medications

11 predominantly, that

12   they reduced protein in the urine. And not only

13 do

14   they use the protein in the urine, they

15 prevented scar

16   tissue forming in the kidney and protected the

17 kidneys.

18   And my colleagues and I published a

19 paper

20   which didn't achieve statistical significance,

21 it was

1   retrospective, but there was a large number of

2 children

3   who were treated either with -- with focal

4 sclerosis,

1   not minimal change, focal sclerosis, who were

2 treated

3   either with the usual poisons like Prednisone

4 and

5   Prograf or Vasotec, the blood pressure

6 medication

7   alone, and we showed there was really no

8 difference in

9   the outcome. In fact, the children who received

10 the

11   Vasotec had a trend towards the statistical

12   significance over the others and fewer side

13 effects.

14   So there is an example where all of

15 our

16   thinking changed from using very

17 immunosuppressive

18   agents, so-called, to using much less toxic

19 agents

20   which have other side -- other effects on the

21 kidney.

1   Do you know what I'm saying?

2   SPECIAL MASTER MILLMAN: Yeah, I do.

3 Thank

4   you.

5   Mr. Wishard.

6   MR. WISHARD: Thank you, ma'am.

7 BY MR. WISHARD:

8   Q.   I want to switch gears and talk a

9 little bit

10   now about JM.

11   A.   Yeah.

12   Q.   And -- and your -- and you did

13 summarize in

14   your first report your thoughts on his medical

15 history.

16   That's Exhibit A at 1 through 3. I'm not going

17 to go

18   into that in detail, but let me ask you a few

19   questions.

1   Do you agree that JM in September of

2   2007 was diagnosed with nephrotic syndrome?

3   A.   Yes, I agree.

4   Q.   And do you agree that his nephrotic

5 syndrome

6   was the form of minimal change nephrotic

7 syndrome or

8   minimal change disease?

9   A.   In retrospect because it was proven by

10   biopsy. And also, because he was steroid

11 sensitive, so

12   he did fulfill criteria for minimal change, yes.

13   Q.   And when he first saw -- started

14 treating

15   with Dr. Seikaly in September of 2007, Dr.

16 Seikaly did

17   some testing for -- one being his creatinine

18   concentrations and levels.

19   Any significance to that -- to what

20 was found

21   there from Dr. Seikaly's testing?

1   A.   So normally for -- for really

2 complicated

3   reasons, which I don't think you want me to

4 spend the

5   day explaining, the -- these glomeruli in

6 minimal

7   change nephrotic syndrome that although they are

8   leaking protein, i.e., albumin, they're actually

9   hyperfunctioning. They're working much harder

10 than

11   normal.

12   So let's say if a normal patient, not

13 a sick

14   patient, had a -- a GFR, which is the filtration

15 rate

16   of 100 percent, the child with minimal change

17 nephrotic

1   syndrome may have 150 or 200 percent GFR. And

2 it's to

3   do with the fact that there's decreased protein

4 in the

5   blood and other factors in the kidney. The

6 results of

7   that is that the serum creatinine, which is

8 normally

9   filtered by the glomerulus and excreted by the

10 kidney,

11   tends to be very low in children with minimal

12 change

13   nephrotic syndrome. It may be .1 or .2 or .4.

14   In the case of JM, when he came into

15 the

16   hospital that time, it was about .8 or .9 and it

17 grows

18   to 1.6 which is quite high. So by definition,

19 by

20   anybody's definition, he had developed acute

21 renal

1   failure, ARF. Or the new terminology is acute

2 renal

3   injury. And acute renal injury or acute renal

4 failure

5   can be caused by a decrease in the blood volume

6 or

7   damage to the kidney or a blockage to the

8 outflow of

9   urine.

10   And in the case of -- of JM, I accept

11   Dr. Quan's view in retrospect that the main

12 reason for

13   this must have been the fact that JM must have

14   been really very volume depleted from vomiting,

15   diarrhea, and also loss of albumin in his urine.

16 I

17   accept that. However, he didn't -- he took a

18 long

19   time, his creatinine came down to .8, .9, but it

20 didn't

21   come down to the levels we normally see. And I

1 would

2   be very concerned about a patient with first

1   presentation of nephrotic syndrome whose

2 creatinine was

3   that high and did not turn to normal. That

4 would

5   really worry me.

6   Q.   The records also show that JM was

7   prescribed first Norvasc and then atenolol.

8   In terms of patients with nephrotic

9 syndrome,

10   which we would later learn is minimal change, is

11 that

12   part of the treatment regimen?

13   A.   It tells me they were really worried

14 about

15   his blood pressure. And they started those

16 medications

17   soon after he presented, relatively soon.

18 Before he

19   had been exposed to a long course of Prednisone

20 or

21   before he gained a lot of weight. So something

1 was

2 going on, because normally in minimal change,

3 the blood

4 pressures are not elevated. Norvasc is a

5 vasodilator.

6 We don't use atenolol anymore, and they used

7 Norvasc.

8 There must have been concerns. But I can't

9 speak for

10 them, but that's my interpretation.

11   Q.   Before we get any further, his

12 nephrotic

13 syndrome, did any -- Dr. Seikaly or any of the

14 treating

15 physicians at the time of his first onset find

16 any type

17 of trigger or cause or virus that may have

18 caused this

19 or did it classify as idiopathic?

20   A.   In the context of this discussion and

21 -- and

1   this case, at no time prior to onset or relapse,

2 did he

1   ever have a high fever or any other features of

2 what

3   you were getting at, this acute innate response.

4 He

5   had nothing like that. He did what a large

6 number of

7   nephrotics do, they just present out of the blue

8   without any other symptoms. And they are called

9   allergies. People say, Oh, you have an allergy.

10   Q.   Similar to Ms. Green who ten years

11 later saw

12   you in a deli and --

13   A.   Yeah.

14   Q.   Now, I think in Dr. Quan's records and

15 maybe

16   in his reports and maybe yesterday, he talked

17 about the

18   fact that, in his view, he thought that JM

19   responded promptly to Prednisone initially.

20   Do you agree with that?

21   A.   Well, I wasn't there, Mr. Wishard, and

1   Special Master, but on 10/11 -- may I read the

2 record

3   that I have here? This is my --

4   SPECIAL MASTER MILLMAN: Yes.

5   THE WITNESS: It's page 2. It's --

6   SPECIAL MASTER MILLMAN: Exhibit A.

7   MR. WISHARD: Exhibit A.

8   THE WITNESS: Exhibit A, yes.

9   SPECIAL MASTER MILLMAN: Yes, I'm

10 there.

11   THE WITNESS: On 10/11/2007, his

12 pediatric

13   nephrologist Mouin G. Seikaly, M.D., noted that

14 JM

1   -- "JM is a patient with new onset nephrotic

2   syndrome who unfortunately had a moderate amount

3 of

4   proteinuria at this visit. He has not completed

5 a full

6   six weeks of daily steroid therapy."

7   And then on 11/7, JM continued to have

8   proteinuria. I agree he did not have nephrotic

9 range

10   proteinuria, but he did not go into -- into

11 remission

12   as defined by the absence of protein in his

13 urine. He

14   continued to have proteinuria despite being on

15   Prednisone for a long time. And he was on 40

16   milligrams every other day, and so he was

17 spilling

18   protein and the Prednisone was not holding him.

19 Weird

20   terms to use, but that's what we say.

21   So Dr. Seikaly expressed the concern

1   that he

2   may -- might relapse once the Prednisone is

3   tapered.

4   And he noted that they discussed the use of

5   Tacrolimus

6   and CellCept therapy and noted that it would be

7   in

8   JM's best interest to start CellCept if he does

9   not tolerate tapering of steroids. And, in

10 fact, he --

11   he -- he was tapered very slowly. Current

12 management

13   of nephrotic syndrome is to reduce the exposure

14 risk to

15   our patients. And there are protocols which

16 give four

17   weeks of this dose and four weeks of that dose

18 and then

19   stop the Prednisone. And the idea of giving a

20 five- or

21   six-month course of Prednisone tells me as a

1 pediatric

1   nephrologist that this doctor was having other

2 sorts of

3   thoughts because of the way that JM was behaving

4   in his first episode.

5   And then he --

6   SPECIAL MASTER MILLMAN: Does that

7 indicate

8   there's something more serious about JM's

9 minimal

10   change disease from the very beginning that

11 would be

12   unusual?

13   THE WITNESS: Well, when I read his

14 case, I

15   was concerned that JM might have a form of

16   nephrotic syndrome that might be more serious.

17 But

18   any -- anything that's been used to try to

19 predict

20   what's going to happen is only -- it's like the

21 polls

1   in the lost election. You -- you take them as

2 you see

3   them. So people could say, well, if somebody

4 has a

5   long course before remission and -- or hematuria

6 or

7   this or that, it might mean that he's going to

8 have a

9   worse course. And that's what they were

10 thinking.

11   He belied that prediction by the fact

12 that

13   when he relapsed the first time, he behaved in a

14   reasonable way as one hopes a nephrotic would

15 behave.

16   And, in fact, he didn't relapse for a long time.

17 His

18   first relapsed was some time after his first

19 episode.

20   So I can waffle about this all sorts of ways

21 because

1   it's -- yes.

1   SPECIAL MASTER MILLMAN: You can only

2   speak -- you're the expert. That's why you're

3 here.

4   THE WITNESS: Yes.

5   SPECIAL MASTER MILLMAN: So if you

6 say, you

7   know, you can't tell how serious or not serious

8 albumin

9   change, nephrotic syndrome is not the same, but

10 you

11   don't know what you've got.

12   THE WITNESS: You put the words in my

13 mouth,

14   ma'am.

15   SPECIAL MASTER MILLMAN: That's fine.

16 Go

17   ahead.

18   MR. WISHARD: Thank you.

19 BY MR. WISHARD:

20   Q.   You mentioned the first relapse which

21 did

1   occur in June of --

2   A.   2009.

3   Q.   -- 2009.   Between the initial onset

4 and the

5   first relapse, JM got a flu vaccination on

6   November 19, 2008.

7   And in your review of the records, did

8 you

9   see anything in the records that would indicate

10 that

11   JM had any type of adverse reaction to that flu

12   vaccination, either locally, fever, swelling or

13   anything?

14   A.   No, sir.

1   Q.   Now, he had his first relapse in June

2 of

3   2009.   And in your view, that's -- that actually

4 was an

5   extended period of time, in -- in -- that he was

6 in

7   remission for.

8   A.   May -- maybe not in the family's view,

9 but it

10   was a nice period.

11   Q.   And he was also -- during this period

12 of time

13   after he got off of Cozaar up until the time he

14 had his

15   first relapse -- or was off of Prednisone, he

16 was on

17   additional antihypertensives.

18   He was on Cozaar; correct?

19   A.   Yeah.

20   Q.   Now, I want to go from the first

21 relapse in

1   June of 2009 up until the time that JM stopped

2   taking Prednisone, which I think was in

3   mid-September 2009, according to the dad's

4   calendar and

5   also the medical records from Dr. Seikaly.

6   You had a chance to review the

7   calendar that

8   was produced by petitioner regarding the

9   readings that

10   were taken from JM from September, I think, 16,

11   2009, up through the day before vaccination, the

12   day of

13   vaccination, before he got the vaccine and the

14   day

15   after?

16   A.   Yes, sir.

17   Q.   And if you -- if you need it, I can

18   provide

1   it. Okay.

2   SPECIAL MASTER MILLMAN: Exhibit 15.

3   MR. WISHARD: Exhibit 15. Thank you,

4   ma'am.

5   BY MR. WISHARD:

6   Q.   In terms of the finding of a weight

7   gain on

8   the morning of the vaccination, a 5-pound weight

9   gain,

10 what significance does that have to you in terms

11 of

12 looking at JM's case and giving your opinions in

13 this proceeding regarding whether the vaccine

14 aggravated his condition?

15   A.   Before I answer that question, I would

16 like

17 to quote what Mr. Miles said about how these

18 values

19 were obtained and who recorded them. And Mr.

20 Miles

21 told us in testimony that he would -- and I

1 believe

2   it's in the record, because I wrote it down,

3 that he

4   would check JM's urine each morning at around

5   7:00, 7:30, 7:30, for -- for protein. He used

6   Multistix, and that he followed the usual

7 procedures of

8   waiting for the usual number of seconds to see

9 if it

10   turned green or not, and then compare the value

11 with

12   the scale on the bottle. And that he also

13 measured

14   JM's blood pressure and his weight.

15   What -- what I found quite striking is

16 that

17   on -- on Wednesday, the 30th of September 2009,

18   JM's weight was 119 pounds and the next day, on

1   the Thursday, it was 124 pounds. And there's a

2 stroke

3   which indicates there was no protein in the

4 urine. And

5   the day after, his weight was 125 pounds with

6 three

7   plus protein and 126 pounds with four plus

8 protein.

9   And I have graphed this just roughly. And what

10 one can

11   see is that from August the 1st to September --

12 sorry,

13   October the 1st, September the 30th, his weight

14 was

15   remarkably stable.

16   SPECIAL MASTER MILLMAN: You're

17 talking from

18   when to when?

19   THE WITNESS: From the first recording

20 of the

21   first page on August the 1st --

1   SPECIAL MASTER MILLMAN: Right, that's

2   Exhibit 15, page 1.

3   THE WITNESS: It was remarkably --

4   SPECIAL MASTER MILLMAN: Page 2. I'm

5   sorry.

6   I'm on the wrong page. One moment. We're in

7   August?

8   Are we in August? Did you say August? Thank

9   you.

10   THE WITNESS: The beginning of August.

11   SPECIAL MASTER MILLMAN: That's page 1

12   of

13   Exhibit 15.

14   THE WITNESS: Yeah, then if you go to

15   page --

16   page 2 of the exhibit, you'll see on September

17   the

18   30th, his weight is actually still in the same

19   ballpark. He's actually around 119. It's been

20   very

1   stable. It's fluctuated a little bit, but it's

2 very

3   stable. And then the next day, it's 124 pounds,

4 which

5   is a 5-pound weight gain which is equivalent to

6 more

7   than 2 liters of fluid retention.

8   And 2 liters of fluid retention is the

9 cutoff

10   used in adults before which or under which you

11 won't

12   see edema. Above 2 liters, you start to see

13 edema,

14   because adults sort of partition the fluid in

15 such a

16   way that they can hide it. But he has this

17 sudden

18   increase in weight.

19   And the weight does not go down the

20 next day.

21   It actually is 125 the next day, 126, 126, 127.

1 In

2   other words, something changed on that

3 particular day

4   that remains constant for the next few days.

5 And then

6   he begins to increase even more as his

7 proteinuria

8   continues.

9   To a nephrologist, this can only mean

10 one

11   thing: that something has changed in his

12 ability to

13   excrete fluid. Given the fact that he's in a

14 nephrotic

15   syndrome, this suggests to me that he was in

16 relapse.

17   SPECIAL MASTER MILLMAN: Does that

18 mean he's

19   in relapse before he took the flu vaccination on

20   October 1st, 2009, which according to, I guess

21 it was

1   Mr. Miles' testimony, was around 3:30 or 4:00

2 p.m.?

3   THE WITNESS: Yes, ma'am. And -- and

4 here's

1   the thing, here's what I want to say. I'm

2 agreeing

3   that that's my answer to you. But these notes

4 are

5   incredibly neat. Mr. Miles says that his wife

6 kept the

7   record. For some reason, he did the testing and

8 the

9   weighing and the blood pressures, but his wife

10 took the

11   record. And then Mr. Miles says that, well,

12 maybe the

13   weight wasn't from early morning. Maybe it was

14 done

15   later in the day. Maybe he -- maybe he --

16   SPECIAL MASTER MILLMAN: Was wearing

17 clothes

18   and shoes.

19   THE WITNESS: Yeah, maybe it was

20 different

21   scale and a different part of the home. So to

1 that, I

2 have this to say: It is my basic principle to

3 believe

4 what people tell me until I can prove otherwise.

5 And

6 giving Mr. Miles the benefit of my doubt, I

7 might say

8 it's possible he was weighed later in the day.

9   SPECIAL MASTER MILLMAN: So it is or

10 is not

11 your testimony that Miles' relapse occurred

12 before his

13 vaccination?

14   THE WITNESS: Yes, ma'am, because the

15 weight

16 went up. And it's possible looking at the

17 weight he

18 would have us look at it, that there was no

19 protein in

20 the morning, that during that day he began to

21 gain

1   weight. We don't know what time he was weighed

2 that

3   day. We've not been told what time he was

4 weighed,

1   that he was already relapsing, that he was one

2 of these

3   children who has an explosive relapse, a very

4 rapid

5   relapse. And that by the next day, he already

6 had the

7   protein in the urine with the same weight. And

8 that

9   this change in his condition occurred prior to

10 him

11   getting the vaccine or even contemporaneously

12 with

13   getting the vaccine, but certainly not a week or

14 six

15   weeks later as has been shown or demonstrated in

16 those

17   few case reports that we were shown yesterday.

18   SPECIAL MASTER MILLMAN: Yesterday,

19 and I

20   forget who said this, it may have been more than

21 one

1   person, but the gist was that no, no, no, even

2 if it's

3   a 5-pound weight gain before the vaccination,

4 you can't

5   count that as a relapse until you see protein

6 spilling

7   in the urine. And since there was no protein

8 when he

9   was tested in his urine on October 1st, that

10 couldn't

11   be the day that he started his relapse. It had

12 to be

13   October 2nd, the next day, because it was plus

14 three.

15   Do you agree with that?

16   THE WITNESS: One could make that

17 argument.

18   One could make that argument. However, if

19 you'll

20   excuse the pun, it doesn't really carry water.

21   SPECIAL MASTER MILLMAN: Because?

1   THE WITNESS: Because he gained 5-

2 pounds.

3   And -- and that's 2 liters of fluid and it was a

4 sudden

1   increase. And I'm offering a way of accepting

2 that

3   maybe he didn't have protein in his urine that

4 morning,

5   but his weight was measured later in that day,

6 either

7   before or after he got the flu vaccine. And by

8 that

9   time, his weight had significantly increased,

10 and it is

11   a significant increase.

12   SPECIAL MASTER MILLMAN: You have to

13 be

14   before the microphone and not ahead of the

15 microphone.

16   THE WITNESS: Sorry. It's a

17 significant

18   increase, ma'am. It would not be a significant

19   increase if we had been seeing that kind of

20 fluctuation

21   in the --

1   SPECIAL MASTER MILLMAN: Up and down.

2   THE WITNESS: Yes, ma'am.

3   SPECIAL MASTER MILLMAN: And you don't

4 see an

5   up-and-down fluctuation for the rest of the

6 month of

7   October. He goes from 124 to 147 by October

8 29th.

9   THE WITNESS: Yes, ma'am.

10   SPECIAL MASTER MILLMAN: So that has

11   significance to you as a pediatric nephrologist.

12   THE WITNESS: Yes.

13   SPECIAL MASTER MILLMAN: And what is

14 the

15   significance?

16   THE WITNESS: The significance is that

17 he has

18   been placed on steroids, and steroids has this

1   unfortunate side effect of causing tremendous

2   increasing appetite, and it also has a side

3 effect of

4   causing salt retention, and the combination of

5 the

6   increase of appetite, the salt retention results

7 in an

8   increase in weight, which is what one would

9 expect.

10   SPECIAL MASTER MILLMAN: My

11 recollection --

12   THE WITNESS: And -- sorry, ma'am.

13   SPECIAL MASTER MILLMAN: Go ahead.

14   THE WITNESS: He had not gone into

15 remission.

16   He was still accumulating fluid.

17   SPECIAL MASTER MILLMAN: All right.

18 And you

19   can certainly explain this in ways that I --

20 even I can

21   think of, but I don't think he went back to Dr.

1 Seikaly

2   until October 9th, and that was when he was put

3 on

4   Prednisone. So you've got a weight increase

5 from

6   October 1st straight through to the 9th. He

7 went from

8   124 pounds to 132 on the 9th or 130 on the 8th.

9 So

10   that increase is part and parcel of the spilling

11 of the

12   urine, the relapse. And from then on he gained

13 even

14   more weight because you're saying he was put on

15 the

16   steroids.

17   THE WITNESS: Absolutely.

18   SPECIAL MASTER MILLMAN: All right.

19   Mr. Wishard.

20   Let me ask you because although I'm

21 jumping

1   into your direct 5,000 times, when would you

2 like to

3   break for lunch? You do not have to break now.

4 You

5   can break in a half an hour, if you want. But

6 you may

7   have some ideas about how you'd like to proceed,

8 so I

9   thought I'd ask.

10   MR. WISHARD: I'll go a half hour,

11 maybe till

12   12:30, and I think I might be done.

13   SPECIAL MASTER MILLMAN: Okay. No

14 problem.

15   MR. WISHARD: If we could. Thank you,

16 ma'am.

17   BY MR. WISHARD:

18   Q.   And getting back, just before we leave

19 the

20   calendar in terms of trends, Dr. Quan said he

21 looked at

1   trends yesterday.

2   Is it fair to say that at least from

3   August 1st up through September 30th, in terms

4 of

5   JM's trend for weight, it was, as you said you

6   mapped out, charted out, consistent.

7   A.   Yes.

8   Q.   And then starting on October 1st, not

9 getting

10   into when that day the weight was taken, but

11 that's

12   when the trend changed in JM's weight?

13   A.   As -- as they say in -- in the lab or

14 in

15   statistical studies, there was a break in the

16 line.

17   There was a definite break in the line.

18   Q.   Okay. And in your view, the

19 vaccination that

1   JM got on October 1st, 2009, 3:00, 4:00 o'clock

2 in

3   the afternoon, did it have any -- did it in

4 anyway

5   aggravate or significantly aggravate his

6 nephrotic

7   syndrome that he suffered before he got the

8   vaccination?

9   A.   After he relapsed that specific time -

10 - that

11   episode, it wasn't easy to get him back into

12 remission.

13   And he was biopsied and he was put on to Prograf

14 and he

15   eventually came off the Prograf. He --

16   Q.   Can we stop a second. Let's talk a

17 little

18   bit about the biopsy.

19   A.   Yes.

20   Q.   What did the biopsy show? Did the

21 biopsy

1   show any damage to the kidney? That was done in

2 May of

3   2010, so it would have been nine-plus months

4 after the

5   vaccination.

6   A.   The biopsy showed minimal change

7 nephrotic

8   syndrome with absolutely no changes except what

9 one

10   would expect.

11   Q.   Okay. I'm sorry. Then you were

12 talking

13   about the Prograf.

14   A.   And once the decision had been made to

15 put

16   him onto Prograf, I would personally think of

17 this in

18   my patients as akin to putting a diabetic onto

19 insulin.

20   And I would be afraid to stop the Prograf,

21 because

1   stopping the Prograf in a significant percentage

2 of

3   cases could result in a relapse in a patient

4 who's on

5   Prograf. Worse than that, in a substantial

6 number of

7   cases, they could become resistant to steroids

8 after

9   the Prograf had been stopped, and I don't know

10 why this

11   occurs. So I was always afraid to stop the

12 Prograf and

13   would continue the Prograf for several years.

14 And

15   Dr. Quan himself said yesterday that he might

16 have

17   preferred to have gone for two years with the

18 Prograf,

19   and that's in his testimony.

20   It is true that after the vaccine, but

21 I do

1   not believe because of the vaccine, it was more

2   difficult to maintain him in remission. That is

3 true.

4   That the vaccine did that, I don't believe.

5   Subsequently, he came off treatment. He was in

6   remission for a while. Not a long period. He

7 then

8   relapsed and had a stroke. And yet he went back

9 into

10   remission in a fairly reasonable time without

11 too much

12   difficulty and has remained in remission for

13 many

14   years, at least five years.

15   So if we look at the totality of this

16 case,

17   from the day he first presented -- I'm sorry. I

18 don't

19   mean to call him a case -- of the totality of JM

20   from the day he first presented till today, he

21 had

1   difficulties in his first episode.   He had

2 difficulties

1   after his second relapse. He had the un --

2 terrible,

3   unfortunate complication of the stroke. And

4 then he

5   has remained in remission, off all treatment.

6 So it is

7   very hard for me to see, in answer to the

8 question, did

9   the --

10   Q.   Actually it was my question.

11   A.   Yes. No, I know it's your question.

12 Well,

13   it's everybody's question: Did the vaccine

14 alter the

15   course of his disease? I cannot look at the

16 course of

17   his disease in -- in choosing one little period

18 of this

19   disease. I have to say this boy has done as

20 well or

21   better than most of my patients have ever done.

1   I hope that answers your question,

2   Mr. Wishard.

3   Q.   It did.   It did.

4   I want to -- there are a couple of

5   things,

6   and I think we covered some of them, from

7   Dr. Bellanti's slides yesterday that you had

8   wanted to

9   comment on.   Let me just look at my notes, and

10 I'm

11 sorry about the delay.   I think you talked about

12 this

13 briefly, but I'm just going to raise it just to

14 make

15 sure.

16   Yesterday during Dr. Bellanti's

17 testimony, he

18 talked about searching for the truth and -- and

19 brought

20 up a few case reports of nephrotic syndrome

21 regarding

1 adults and also mentioned that minimal change

2 disease

3 is the same in kids and adults.

4 Do you have any comments about that?

5 A. Just repeat the last part of that

6 sentence.

7 Q. Sure. The last part of my statement

8 was: I

9 think there was a statement that minimal change

10 disease

11 is the same in children and adults.

12 SPECIAL MASTER MILLMAN: Was that "is

13 not"?

14 MR. WISHARD: Is.

15 SPECIAL MASTER MILLMAN: Is? Because

16 Dr. Quan testified that it's totally different

17 when

18 you're dealing with adults than with children.

19 BY MR. WISHARD:

20 Q. Okay. Let me ask you, then: Is

21 minimal

1   change disease in adults the same as it is in

2   children,

3   in your view?

4   A.   So in about 1970-something when I was

5   doing

6   adult nephrology, there was a brilliant paper in

7   the

8   Quarterly Journal of Medicine, which used to be

9   prestigious from England, in which they asked

10   this

11   question.   The reason they asked this question

12   was

13   because most children with nephrotic syndrome

14   minimal

15   change respond to steroids and they respond

16   within

17   about two weeks usually, whereas most adults had

18   difficulty responding to steroids.   And so the

1   legitimate question that was raised was: Are

2 these two

3   different conditions?   Or are they behaving

4 differently

5   because of age?

6   What these people did was to look at

7 the

8   dosing of Prednisone, and the dosing of

9 Prednisone is

10   really quite interesting because I don't know

11 any other

12   medication that's dosed the way Prednisone's

13 dosed.

14   The dose of Prednisone is 2 milligrams per kilo

15 up to

16   30 kilos.   So if you're 30 kilos which is about

17   70 pounds, you will get 60 milligrams of

18 Prednisone.

19   But if you're 100 kilos or 200 kilos, they might

20 push

21   you up to 90 milligrams of Prednisone.   They

1 would be

2   afraid to give you 2 kilo -- like 200 milligrams

3 a day

4   or 300 milligrams a day because of the side

5 effects.

6   And they did this study, which was

7 very

8   brave, where they gave their patients what they

9 thought

10   would be the appropriate dose that was upscaled

11 for

12   their weight. And those patients went into

13 remission.

14   But of course they had terrible side effects.

15 And

16   that -- that is a dilemma that is very difficult

17 to

18   deal with. But if we think about it, any

19 patient up to

20   30 kilos gets a maximum of 60 milligrams a day,

21 but if

1   that child's 40 kilos, 50 kilos, 90 kilos, still

2 be

3   getting 60 milligrams a day.

4   And that is possibly one of the

5 reasons we

1   see steroid resistance in some of our patients,

2 that

3   we're not really dosing them appropriately. And

4 I

5   don't want to talk about it out of context of JM

6   but just philosophically. And that's why we

7 started to

8   give intravenous Solu-Medrol which is a form of

9   steroid, very high doses, but very quickly and

10 not for

11   a long time to try to get them into remission.

12   So do I think that minimal change

13 nephrotic

14   syndrome is different in adults versus children?

15 I

16   don't think there's any real evidence that it's

17   different.

18   Q.   Okay.

19   A.   Surely -- no, I don't think there's

20 any

21   evidence.

1   Q.   Okay. We had talked earlier this

2 morning and

3   yesterday about several pages of Dr. Bellanti's

4 slide

5   show, and I think we covered it, but I just want

6 to

7   cover -- I just want to make sure that you've

8 covered

9   the points in your discussion today. This is

10   Exhibit 100. I'm looking at pages 40 and 41.

11   Is there anything in addition --

12 sorry. I

13   have to speak up here.

14   Is there anything in addition that you

15 want

16   to include in your testimony today? I know you

17   testified about some of the issues involved on

18 these

1   slides.

2   A.   So -- so Dr. Bellanti in this table or

3   slide

4   has listed three mechanisms of glomerular

5   injury. The

6   third is mutations in the podocyte or slit

7   diaphragm

8   proteins which I've talked about. And I agree

9   with

10   that, except that this can appear in adults as

11   well.

12   And of course, the whole concept of circulating

13   antigen-antibody complexes, which is very

14   problematical, because there is no real evidence

15   that

16   circulating antigen-antibody complement

17   complexes are

18   causative of the damage that occurs in

19   glomerular

20   nephritis.

21   And the reason I say this is because

1   Dr. Couser, whose paper has been quoted, did

2 some

3   extraordinary studies in membranous

4 glomerulopathy in

5   which he said a patient who has circulating

6 complexes

7   depending on the size Type 1, Type 2, Type 3,

8 that

9   these complexes will either be so big they'll be

10 taken

11   up by the liver and spleen and the lymph nodes,

12 or so

13   small they'll just pass into the urine, or of a

14 size

15   that we see in the glomerulus. But these

16 complexes

17   form on the other side of the basement membrane.

18 And

19   somehow these complexes have to be able to get

20 through

21   a basement membrane and form these big chunks on

1 the

2   other side of the basement membrane.

1   And so he predicted that what is

2 happening is

3   that there is an in situ antigen in the basement

4   membrane and that this accumulates

5 immunoglobulins and

6   complement that can pass through the membrane

7 and that

8   this results in the formation of these complexes

9 which

10   either attract phagocytes or they damage the

11 podocytes.

12   And in recent years, Dr. Salant from

13 Boston

14   has been able -- with his group has been able to

15 show

16   exactly what is happening, that in this

17 membranous GN,

18   the idiopathic form where there's no apparent

19 cause,

20   like thyroid disease or hepatitis B, that

21 there's a

1   PLA2R. It's called Phospholipase A2 Receptor

2 antigen

3   that's in the membrane, and that this somehow

4 becomes

5   exposed, and this is what results in the

6 formation of

7   the complex. This triggers the -- the formation

8 of the

9   complex. So there I don't agree completely with

10   Dr. Bellanti's formulation because that is quite

11 an old

12   formulation.

13   And then in the case of minimal change

14   disease, he has said that there are circulating

15 factors

16   in minimal change disease and primary focal

17 sclerosis

18   glomerulus sclerosis which he says he thinks is

19 the

20   reason why these patients have proteinuria.

21   Q.   Which is the next page you're talking

1 about

2   now?

1   A.   Yeah.   But it's the first thing he

2 listed,

3   and it's the next page.   The problem is, and

4   Dr. Levinson can speak to this better than I

5 can,

6   the -- the music that is made by these factors

7 that are

8   being found is atonal.   This is not Beethoven or

9   Mozart.   There is no patent.   There is no -- it

10 is so

11   jumbled, it is so atonal as to make no sense

12   whatsoever.

13   SPECIAL MASTER MILLMAN: What makes no

14 sense?

15   What has no patterns?

16   THE WITNESS: The cytokines that go up

17 and

18   the cytokines that go down and the T cells that

19 do this

20   and the T cells that do that, which is the

21 circulating

1   factors that he's talking about.

2   SPECIAL MASTER MILLMAN: Well, I need

3 a

4   little more explanation.

5   THE WITNESS: Yes.

6   SPECIAL MASTER MILLMAN: Doctor, when

7   Dr. Bellanti was on yesterday afternoon and he

8 was

9   explaining the difference between the innate and

10 the

11   adaptive --

12   THE WITNESS: Yeah.

13   SPECIAL MASTER MILLMAN: -- immune

14 systems,

15   and he said of course, this one day -- because

16 he's

17   reviewing this as a one-day onset of remission.

18 He

1   says, Well, you have cytokines. And I said,

2 Where is

3   the inflammation? He had no fever, no systemic

4   anything. And he said, No, that doesn't matter.

5 I

6   kind of get lost after that. But nevertheless,

7   cytokines are supposed to be produced. In other

8 words,

9   if you're going to stimulate the immune system

10 to

11   produce antibodies to the antigen that you've

12 received

13   from the injection, this is normal. It doesn't

14 mean

15   it's -- it's disease producing.

16   And so my understanding what you just

17 said is

18   that there is no direct effect like you might be

19 able

20   to follow a Mozart symphony because it has a

21 pattern

1   and you -- you can understand the different

2 movements

3   in the production of cytokines.

4   Have I got that right so far?

5   THE WITNESS: Perfectly.

6   SPECIAL MASTER MILLMAN: Whereas if

7 you take

8   Phillip Glass or any of the others who do not

9 create --

10   if you're saying you -- you don't want to listen

11 to

12   that, but if you like it to be a little

13 confused, you

14   can listen to -- it's atonal. The cytokines do

15   whatever they do and there is no pattern and,

16   therefore, they cannot be a connection between

17 the

18   production of cytokines which is a result of the

19   vaccination and the remission which is

20 occurring,

1   minimal change nephrotic syndrome.

2   Have I got that right?

3   THE WITNESS: Absolutely.

4   MR. WISHARD: You said remission. Did

5 you

6   mean relapse, ma'am? I'm sorry.

7   THE WITNESS: It's relapse.

8   SPECIAL MASTER MILLMAN: Did I say

9 remission?

10   Thank you. I tell you we all need each other.

11   MR. WISHARD: Yes, ma'am.

12   SPECIAL MASTER MILLMAN: Okay. I

13 meant

14   relapse.

15   THE WITNESS: Yes, ma'am.

16   SPECIAL MASTER MILLMAN: It's not

17 remission

18   because he's starting up again. Now I

19 understand.

20   Did you complete what you wanted to

21 say?

1   THE WITNESS: No, but you -- you laid

2 the

3   groundwork for my problem which is his graphic

4   description of the innate process and then the

5 adaptive

6   mechanisms, which if -- to be generous, if he

7 were

8   talking about membranous GN or lupus or

9   post-streptococcal glomerulonephritis, I could

10 say,

11   hmm. I can see this is -- this is possible.

12 But what

13   he's describing in the context of this disease

14 that I

15   have taken care of for 50 years, they are not

16   superimposable upon each other.

1   SPECIAL MASTER MILLMAN: You mean

2 "they" by

3   cytokines and --

4   THE WITNESS: Absolutely. His scheme

5 --

6   schema and his speculations, which he admits are

7   speculations, I can quote him. He -- he wrote

8 and said

9   that this is theory in response to one of my

10 critiques.

11   Whether it is or isn't, there is no evidence of

12 any of

13   this happening in the way that he is saying in

14 children

15   with nephrotic syndrome of the minimal change

16 variety.

17   And I think what -- what also happened

18 was

19   that other articles were thrown in somehow to

20 support

21   this. The one I chose to talk about today is

1   Dr. Dickinson's article --

2   BY MR. WISHARD:

3   Q.   Which is actually -- was one of the

4 articles

5   on the PowerPoint which we don't have a copy of

6 yet,

7   but we do have the abstract, which I haven't

8 marked or

9   anything yet because I just pulled up the

10 abstract this

11   morning, the full abstract not just the piece

12 that was

13   put on the PowerPoint. I can do that now.

14   A.   And in this article, it's entitled

15   "Unraveling the Immunopathogenesis of Glomerular

16   Disease." Now, truthfully I have the abstract.

17 We

18   haven't been able to get the paper.

19   SPECIAL MASTER MILLMAN: Yes, you'll

20 have the

1   opportunity, as I said yesterday.

2   THE WITNESS: But using the abstract,

3 Bonny

4   Dickinson is talking about nephrotic syndrome

5   characterized by the infiltration of

6 inflammatory cells

7   into the mesangium or subendothelium --

8 mesangium is

9   the part of the glomerulus in between the little

10 vessels, kind of like the supporting structure.

11 And so

12 she says nephritic syndrome is characterized by

13 the

14 infiltration of inflammatory cells into the

15 mesangium

16 and subendothelium, whereas nephrotic syndrome

17 is

18 characterized by damage to podocytes driven by

19 immune

20 complexes in the subepithelial space.

21   And -- and what I've said many times

1 today,

2 there is absolutely no evidence for the presence

3 of the

4 immune complexes in the subepithelial space or

5 anywhere

6 else in the kidney in minimal change nephrotic

7 syndrome. So that particular paper does not

8 address

9 what we're talking about. It addresses a

10 totally

11 different syndrome or condition, and I don't

12 think

13 that's -- you cannot extrapolate from one to the

14 other.

15   SPECIAL MASTER MILLMAN: Now, I don't

16 know,

17 because this seems to be in the immunologic

18 sphere, if

19 Dr. Kaplan would like to respond to the other --

20 explanation for how this occurred as an

21 anamnestic

1   response from the November 19th, 2008,

2 vaccination

1   against flu to the October 1st, 2009, because

2 there's

3   only one of the three strains of flu vaccine --

4 virus,

5   sorry, that's different and that having two-

6 thirds of

7   the components being identical would prompt a

8 faster

9   reaction.

10   THE WITNESS: So, Special Master, when

11 I

12   thought I might have to respond to that, I had

13 an acute

14   anaphylactoid reaction.

15   SPECIAL MASTER MILLMAN: You do not

16 have to

17   respond to it.

18   THE WITNESS: No, no.   Fortunately, he

19 who

20   laughs loudest, Dr. Levinson is going to address

21 that

1   as an immunologist.

2   SPECIAL MASTER MILLMAN: Yes.   I just

3   wanted

4   to ask, and it's certainly an immunologic

5   question and

6   Dr. Levinson will deal with that.

7   THE WITNESS: Yeah.

8   SPECIAL MASTER MILLMAN: Okay.   Go

9   ahead,

10 Mr. Wishard.

11 BY MR. WISHARD:

12   Q.   And I think you covered --

13   A.   Yes, I did.

14   Q.   We covered that.   So we don't need to

15 cover

16 that.

17   There were two more articles I think

18 that you

1   wanted to talk about. One --

2   A.   Yes, sir.

3   Q.   -- one authored by Zhu, Z-h-u, which

4   is

5   Exhibit C at Tab 7.

6   Why did you want to raise that article

7   in the

8   context of what you heard yesterday?

9   A.   Special Master, and others, this paper

10 from

11 2009 which I had quoted in my letter is entitled

12 "Association of Influenza Vaccination With the

13 Reduced

14 Risk of Venous Thromboembolism," not just in

15 nephrotic

16 syndrome but in general. And this was done on

17 hundreds

18 and hundreds of adults, those who received the

19 vaccine,

20 those who didn't, and the vaccine significantly

21 -- at a

1   significant level protected those who received

2 the

3   vaccine from developing a clot.

4   And now, they weren't nephrotics, but

5 it

6   protected them. And there has been a suggestion

7 or a

8   reaction that somehow the fact that JM had a

9   relapse in association with the vaccine and then

10 had a

11   stroke 22 months later, that somehow that had to

12 be

13   associated with the vaccine. And that's

14 inconceivable.

15   It is absolutely inconceivable.

16   SPECIAL MASTER MILLMAN: I think

17 petitioner's

18   approach is that if he hadn't had the flu

19 vaccine in

20   2009, he wouldn't have relapsed. If he hadn't

1   relapsed, he wouldn't have been put on steroids

2 and

3   then failed to recover from that. And then he

4 had to

5   be put on Prograf, and it's because of that --

6 this is

7   a tort analysis; torts meaning civil wrongs

8 based on

9   negligence or it could be intentional. Well, we

10 don't

11   need to talk about it.

12   But, anyway, if it hadn't been for

13 this, this

14   wouldn't have happened, that wouldn't have

15 happened,

16   and that wouldn't have happened. So you get to

17 the

18   stroke part 22 months later because of this

19 series of

20   events that happened.

21   THE WITNESS: So that's very

1 Aristotelian, as

2 Dr. Bellanti was trying to tell us about A to B

3 to C.

4 And life isn't Aristotelian. Certainly biology

5 isn't.

6 Biology is now a shower of arrows. There is no

7 direct

8 Path A for anything anymore. Well, maybe there

9 are

10 some. But look at any diagram and what you see

11 are

12 arrows in every direction doing all kinds of

13 things.

14   And I think, with the greatest

15 respect, to

16 say that because he had the vaccine and relapse

17 and

18 then had another relapse and then had a stroke,

19 that

20 that was the cause -- caused by the vaccine, I

21 think

1   that's inconceivable.   That's not based on

2 anything

3   that -- that can be somehow made into a coherent

4   scientific story.   It just doesn't make sense.

1   SPECIAL MASTER MILLMAN: Medically.

2   THE WITNESS: Medically, it doesn't

3 make

4   sense.

5   SPECIAL MASTER MILLMAN: And the

6 reason it

7   doesn't make sense medically is?

8   THE WITNESS: Because, first of all,

9 it's a

10   very long period after he got the vaccine.

11 Secondly,

12   he had responded to treatment and had gone into

13   remission. It's true he subsequently relapsed.

14 We

15   don't know if he would have done that anyhow had

16 he not

17   received the vaccine. I suspect he would have.

18 And

19   then he had another relapse. I don't know where

20 it was

21   because they were talking about a hotel room,

1 and I

2   didn't know --

3   SPECIAL MASTER MILLMAN: In Dallas,

4 Texas.

5   THE WITNESS: Yes, I think I know

6 where that

7   is. Yeah, I've heard of that.

8   And I think that he had this stroke,

9 and it

10   was an arterial stroke. And it -- it bothers me

11   tremendously why a young boy would have an

12 arterial

13   thrombus. And the idea is that it must be

14 related to

15   the nephrotic syndrome because of loss of

16 factors in

17   his urine. In fact, it's extremely rare in the

18   nephrotic syndrome to see this in a child. And

19 -- the

20   arterial thrombus and specifically in the

21 cerebral

1   artery. And I have tried hard to think of what

2 might

3   be -- might have contributed to this leaving

4 aside the

5   vaccine.

6   He -- he had this stroke after being

7 in

8   relapse for a very short time. He didn't really

9 have a

10   chance to lose the massive amounts of

11 procoagulation

12   and anticoagulation factors that people talk

13 about

14   in -- in people who do have venous thrombi. And

15 --

16   SPECIAL MASTER MILLMAN: This is

17 arterial

18   thrombi.

19   THE WITNESS: That's exactly right,

20 which is

21   even more of a problem because it's so rare.

1 And

2   because in a young person, the -- the vessels,

3 unlike

4   in someone my age where they are tortuous and

5 there's

6   plaque and calcium and all kinds of awful stuff

7 and --

8   and blood flow is impeded and clots form in

9 blood

10   vessels and we get strokes and other awful

11 things, this

12   doesn't happen in young people unless something

13 else is

14   going on.

15   So one of the things we thought about

16 was the

17   factor V Leiden, and we could argue about that

18 till the

19   cows come home. The mutation in factor V

20 Leiden, in

21   contradiction to what Dr. Bellanti said, does

1 not cause

2   bleeding. It causes clotting. Not bleeding.

3 But it's

4   problematical, factor V Leiden.

1   What I noticed on the report of the

2 MRA of

3   his head was that he did have a -- they said

4 they

5   thought he had narrowing of his middle cerebral

6 artery,

7   that there was an area that was narrowed. Now,

8 I am

9   not a neuroradiologist. I've written with

10 others quite

11   a number of papers on narrow arteries and why

12 they're

13   so important in terms of stroke and in terms of

14 severe

15   hypertension. But I'm left puzzled as to why he

16 had

17   the -- had the stroke, quite frankly.

18   I cannot ascribe it to the vaccine. I

19 cannot

20   ascribe it even to the nephrotic syndrome in

21 this

1   context because -- I'm sorry I'm repeating

2 myself.

3   SPECIAL MASTER MILLMAN: No, it's

4 fine.

5   THE WITNESS: -- there are hardly any

6 case

7   reports of this. So even if you go and read

8 about it,

9   and I as a nephrologist who -- who -- who worked

10 in all

11   these places and saw all these children for all

12 these

13   years never saw a single case of a cerebral

14 artery

15   thrombus in a child with nephrotic syndrome. So

16 to me,

17   it's an area that needs to be thought about

18 much, much

19   more.

20   SPECIAL MASTER MILLMAN: And you don't

21   ascribe it to the Prograf or taking him off the

1   Prograf?

2   THE WITNESS: I actually did a

3 literature

1   search on that and could find nothing to link

2 the two.

3   SPECIAL MASTER MILLMAN: Were all

4 three

5   strokes in the artery, the same artery, or did

6 the

7   other two vary?

8   THE WITNESS: So I can't answer that

9 with

10   great assurance. Or -- one of the things that

11 really

12   bothered me about his stroke, aside from the

13 things

14   that I've been telling you that bothered me, and

15 I'm

16   being totally honest talking more like a

17 pediatrician

18   than somebody giving witness, is that he had

19 what they

20   described as multiple punctate spots of what

21 looked

1   like infarcts in the other side of his brain.

2 And I

3   couldn't really understand what that was all

4 about.

5   SPECIAL MASTER MILLMAN: Is that in

6 the

7   arteries or something else?

8   THE WITNESS: I don't know. And if he

9 had

10   been my patient, I would have taken his imaging

11 studies

12   to our neurological -- neuroradiological team,

13 who are

14   really amazing. And then they would have given

15 -- and

16   we have a special stroke clinic at the

17 children's

18   hospital where -- where people are seen. And

19 it's -- I

20   don't know the answer. I just don't know. I'm

21 left

1   puzzled by the stroke. That's my honest

2 opinion.

3   SPECIAL MASTER MILLMAN: Are venal

4 strokes

5   more common in children?

1   THE WITNESS: Are what?

2   SPECIAL MASTER MILLMAN: Venal; that

3 is, a

4   stroke in a vein not an artery. Venous.

5   THE WITNESS: Twenty to one.

6   SPECIAL MASTER MILLMAN: And is that

7 related

8   to nephrotic syndrome?

9   THE WITNESS: Not necessarily.

10   SPECIAL MASTER MILLMAN: Okay.

11   THE WITNESS: For example, are you --

12 did you

13   say venous?

14   SPECIAL MASTER MILLMAN: Well, I

15 didn't know

16   what the adjective should be. It could be

17 venal,

18   v-e-n-a-l. Venous, v-e-n-o-u-s. So I thought

19 I'd let

20   you pick.

21   THE WITNESS: I'm sorry. A venous

1 thrombus

2 in the brain usually affects what's called the

3 sagittal

4 sinus. It's part of the brain which isn't --

5 it's

6 draining blood. They don't really get a stroke.

7 It's

8 not the same as an arterial stroke. When you're

9 looking at children who have strokes in their

10 arteries

11 in the brain, you have to think of sickle cell

12 disease.

13 You have to think of a condition called Williams

14 syndrome. My wife takes care of other vascular

15 disorders, neurofibromatosis. There's a long,

16 long

17 list of conditions that have to be looked for to

18 try

1   and account for the stroke. And I don't know

2 exactly

3   what caused it.

4   SPECIAL MASTER MILLMAN: Would it be

5 the

6   Leiden 5 factor mutation?

7   THE WITNESS: I'm going to say that's

8 -- I'm

9   not sure how much that contributed.

10   SPECIAL MASTER MILLMAN: Okay. Thank

11 you.

12   Go ahead.

13   BY MR. WISHARD:

14   Q.   Just one additional article. You had

15   mentioned Greenbaum which is exhibit -- and I

16 think

17   that was part of the PowerPoint as well.

18   A.   Yeah.

19   Q.   I think Exhibit -- Exhibit 7 -- or,

20 excuse

21   me, Exhibit C, page -- Tab 17. I'm going to

1 hand you a

2 copy of that if you don't have it.

3   A.   Dr. Bellanti put up a slide in which

4 he

5 quoted this paper by Greenbaum and Bendorf and

6 Smoyer.

7 And I know Dr. Smoyer because he trained under

8 me, and

9 Dr. Greenbaum I know as well.

10   SPECIAL MASTER MILLMAN: That's S-m-o-

11 y-e-r.

12   THE WITNESS: Yeah.   And in the

13 abstract,

14 Dr. Bellanti -- Bellanti quoted -- and may I

15 read --

16 "These strategies have historically focused on

17 identifying effective alternative

18 immunosuppressant

1   agents such as cyclosporin and Tacrolimus. Yet

2   evidence now indicates that nephrotic syndrome

3 results

4   from podocyte dysfunction. Even conventional

5   immunosuppressant agents such as glucocorticoids

6 and

7   cyclosporin directly affect podocyte structure

8 and

9   function challenging the immune theory of the

10   pathogenesis of childhood nephrotic syndrome in

11 which

12   this disease is caused by T cells."

13   And I -- I only quote this one because

14 I

15   don't believe this challenge to the theory was

16 put up

17   on the screen. And there are several other

18 very, very

19   important papers by workers in the field who

20 also doubt

21   or show or feel that there's no support for

1   immunopathogenesis, cytokine pathogenesis for

2 minimal

3   change nephrotic syndrome.

4   SPECIAL MASTER MILLMAN: I notice that

5 the

6   Greenbaum article was published in AMRA in 2015.

7   So how new is this understanding that

8 a

9   minimal change nephrotic syndrome is not an

10   immune-based disease?

11   THE WITNESS: It's -- I can't say

12 exactly

13   when -- when people changed their minds, but

14 certainly

15   this century.

16   SPECIAL MASTER MILLMAN: It's what?

17   THE WITNESS: In this century.

1   SPECIAL MASTER MILLMAN: Oh, well,

2 that's --

3   that's --

4   THE WITNESS: Maybe -- maybe the last

5 ten

6   years.

7   SPECIAL MASTER MILLMAN: Okay.   This

8 century.

9   THE WITNESS: It's all because of this

10 --

11   this amazing discovery of the mutation of the

12 nephron

13   in congenital nephrotic syndrome which just

14 totally

15   changed the whole view of nephrotic syndrome.

16 So much

17   so, Special Master, that a new term has been

18 coined to

19   describe all these conditions.   And they're now

20 called

21   the podocytopathies.

542

1   SPECIAL MASTER MILLMAN: I'm writing

2 it down.

3   Podocy what?

4   THE WITNESS: Cytopathy.

5   SPECIAL MASTER MILLMAN: Cytopathy.

6 Disease

7   of the foot.

8   THE WITNESS: Of the -- yes, of the

9   podocytes, exactly.

10   SPECIAL MASTER MILLMAN:

11 Podocytopathy, does

12   it only apply to kidneys?

13   THE WITNESS: Beg your pardon?

14   SPECIAL MASTER MILLMAN: Kidneys.

15 Does it

16   only apply to kidney disease? Because there's

17 only

18   podos or feet in kidneys, podocytes.

1   THE WITNESS: Well, the thing about

2 the human

3   body, it's miserably complicated. In Alport

4 syndrome

5   where the glomeruli are affected so badly they

6 need a

7   kidney transplant, parts of the ear are affected

8 as

9   well. And parts of the eye are affected. So

10 there are

11 different organs that are affected depending on

12 what

13 the -- the genetic interactions are on different

14 parts

15 of the body.

16   SPECIAL MASTER MILLMAN: But certainly

17 minimal change nephrotic syndrome would be a

18 podocytopathy, a disease of the podocytes solely

19 in the

20 kidneys --

21   THE WITNESS: Yes, ma'am.

1   SPECIAL MASTER MILLMAN: -- without

2 extension

3   to your ears or your wherever else you were --

4   THE WITNESS: Yes. Yes, ma'am.

5 Except --

6   yes.

7   SPECIAL MASTER MILLMAN: Yes?

8   MR. WISHARD: Just for the record, I

9 thought

10   you said the -- the Greenbaum was 2015. It's

11 actually

12   2012. So it takes it back a couple more years.

13   SPECIAL MASTER MILLMAN: Is it 2012?

14   MR. WISHARD: Yeah.

15   SPECIAL MASTER MILLMAN: I just was

16 looking

17   for the date and I saw Emory 2015.

1   Where is your 2012 in here?

2   MR. WISHARD: It says at the bottom

3 Volume VIII --

4   SPECIAL MASTER MILLMAN: Got it.

5 You're

6 right. Published online 2012. So sorry.

7   MR. WISHARD: So it takes us back a

8 little

9 bit earlier in this century.

10   SPECIAL MASTER MILLMAN: Yes. No, but

11 he

12 said, though, it's the last ten years. So since

13 this

14 is 2017, we can go back to 2007. Thank you.

15   MR. WISHARD: That's all the questions

16 I

17 have. Thank you, Doctor.

18   SPECIAL MASTER MILLMAN: All right.

19 So

20 you're very prompt. It is 12:30. You can run

21 the

1   trains. How's that?

2   MR. WISHARD: No thanks. Especially

3   the

4   Metro.

5   SPECIAL MASTER MILLMAN: No. Well,

6   any --

7   any help for our local subway would be

8   appreciated.

9   Would you like to take a lunch break

10 now?

11   It's 12:30. I assume that Mr. McHugh would like

12 to do

13   a cross-examination of Dr. Kaplan. Would you

14 like to

15   take a break?

16   MR. WISHARD: Yes, Your Honor.

17   SPECIAL MASTER MILLMAN: And how long

18 would

1   you like this break?

2   MR. WISHARD: An hour would be fine.

3   SPECIAL MASTER MILLMAN: Okay. So we

4 will go

5   off the record right now, and we will resume at

6 1:30.

7   Thank you very much. Appreciate that.

8   (Whereupon a lunch recess was

9 taken.)

10   SPECIAL MASTER MILLMAN: Mr. McHugh,

11 we're

12 back on the record.

13   Are you ready to do cross-examination?

14   MR. McHUGH: I am, Your Honor.

15   SPECIAL MASTER MILLMAN: Very well.

16 Thank

17   you.

18

19   CROSS-EXAMINATION

20   BY MR. McHUGH:

21   Q.   Good afternoon, Doctor.

1   A.   Good afternoon, sir.

2   Q.   Going to your Exhibit A, Government's

3   Exhibit A, which is your report of June 18th of

4 2013,

5   and down on page 5, the second to the last

6 paragraph on

7   the page, you state that "There's no scientific

8   evidence that inactivated flu vaccine or any

9 other

10   vaccine causes or participates in nephrotic

11 syndrome or

12   that it or any other vaccine participates in

13 relapse."

14   Is -- is that your testimony?

```
1        A.    That's what I wrote, yes, sir.

2        Q.    That's what you said?

3        A.    Yes, sir.

4        Q.    And you -- you still hold to that?

5        A.    Yes, sir.

6        Q.    Okay.

7              MR. McHUGH:  May we play a --

8              SPECIAL MASTER MILLMAN:  I'm sorry.

9  What is

10   it?

11             MR. McHUGH:  We have to play a video,

12 Your

13   Honor.

14             SPECIAL MASTER MILLMAN:  You want to

15 play a

16   video?

17             MR. McHUGH:  Yes, play a video, very

18 short

19   video.

20             SPECIAL MASTER MILLMAN:  Okay.  I'm

21 sorry.
```

1   What?

2   BY MR. McHUGH:

3   Q.   Doctor, do you remember giving

4 lectures for

5 NephCure?

6   A.   Yes.

7   SPECIAL MASTER MILLMAN: Could you

8 spell

9 NephCure.

10   N-e-p-h-C-u-r-e, NephCure Foundation.

11   SPECIAL MASTER MILLMAN: N-e-p-h?

1   MR. MILES: N-e-p-h, like nephrotic.

2   SPECIAL MASTER MILLMAN: Are you going

3 to

4   submit this into evidence, Mr. McHugh? How do

5 you do

6   that on a CD?

7   MR. McHUGH: I'm not sure.

8   SPECIAL MASTER MILLMAN: It might be

9 on a CD.

10   I bet you Mr. Miles knows.

11   MR. MILES: I'm sorry?

12   SPECIAL MASTER MILLMAN: And Dr.

13 Bellanti

14   would definitely know.

15   MR. McHUGH: Any 12 year old or Mr.

16 Miles.

17   Not me, except that I --

18   SPECIAL MASTER MILLMAN: All right.

19 How --

20   before we get into watching the video, how long

21 is it?

1   MR. MILES: Less than three or four

2 minutes.

3   SPECIAL MASTER MILLMAN: Three to four

4 minutes. Go ahead. I'm looking at the video.

5   MR. WISHARD: Can we raise the volume

6 'cause

7 I couldn't hear it?

8   SPECIAL MASTER MILLMAN: Is there

9 sound in

10 this video?

11   MR. McHUGH: Oh, yes.

12   (Video clip was played.)

13   DR. KAPLAN: Often in the high doses,

14 especially in postpubertal males --

1   (Video clip was stopped.)

2   SPECIAL MASTER MILLMAN: I can't hear

3 it.

4   MR. McHUGH: I can't hear it.

5   SPECIAL MASTER MILLMAN: Could you

6 restart it

7   and --

8   MR. MILES: I can put the volume up.

9   SPECIAL MASTER MILLMAN: Yes, that

10 would help

11   I think.

12   MR. MILES: But it doesn't seem to be

13 going

14   through the video link, so I'm trying to play it

15   through the speaker.

16   SPECIAL MASTER MILLMAN: We have

17 microphones.

18   Can you put a microphone in front of whatever

19   constitutes a speaker on your computer?

20   MR. MILES: That's what I'm trying to

21 do.

1   (Video clip was played.)

2   DR. KAPLAN: And there are a small

3 number of

4   people who have developed malignancies,

5 presumably

6   because of cyclophosphamide.

7   So what -- what we have here is it --

8 it's --

9   it's as if -- as if we are living in an age of

10 jet

11 travel and amazing telecommunications and the

12 Internet

13 and everything, but we still have to engage our

14 homes

15 and use candles for light. We have not had

16 actually

17 significant advance in the treatment of minimal

18 change

1 nephrotic syndrome for about 60 years.   The

2 steroids

3 were discovered by two men who got the Nobel

4 prize.

5 You know, they got it in 19 -- it was the late

6 '50s or

7 early '50s, yeah, early '50s. And Cytoxan was

8 first

9 used during the war. And Cytoxan had been

10 invented by

11 German scientists in the first world war it was

12 called

13 nitrogen mustard, and it was used to gas Allied

14 troops

15 on the Western Front. But somebody used it to

16 treat

17 nephrotic syndrome and it worked. It also was

18 useful

19 for certain kinds of cancer. And all the other

20 things

21 we've tried have not proved to be as useful as

1   Prednisone and maybe Cytoxan or

2 cyclophosphamide.

3   And that's why a clinician like myself

4 feels

5   that the kind of work -- and this is sponsored

6 by

7   Dr. -- by the scientists working in the lab,

8   Dr. Holzman and his colleagues, if they don't

9 find for

10   us some new understanding of the biology of

11 these

12   conditions, it's not clear where we're going to

13 go with

14   these conditions.

15   Having said that, life is very

16 strange.

17 Nobody would ever have predicted that an ACE

18 inhibitor

19   that was -- it was produced by Merck for the

20 treatment

21   of hypertension would become one of the most

1 important

2   medications for the use of people with kidney

3 disease

4   of all kinds. So sometimes there are

5 serendipitous

1   things that happen, and we have to keep our

2 minds open

3   to them.

4   So here I am, I've been a pediatric

5   nephrologist for 36 years since I started, 38

6 years,

7   and I have seen so little advancement in the

8 treatment.

9   On the other hand, I have to say I have seen one

10 child

11   die from who had minimal change nephrotic

12 syndrome, and

13   she died because she developed an infection with

14   pneumococcus, and she died from the pneumococcal

15   infection.

16   And I -- I -- I lost my slide that I

17 had on

18   inoculations. And I just want to end by saying

19 a few

20   words about inoculations. I have been worried

21 about

1   inoculating kids with nephrotic syndrome because

2 it may

3   increase the relapse rate. And indeed, Dr.

4 Trumpatine

5   in London has shown recently that using the new

6   meningococcal vaccine, patients who got that

7   meningococcal vaccine had an increased relapse

8 rate in

9   the subsequent 12 months compared to the

10 previous 12

11   months.

12   And now I have to say: So what? I

13 have seen

14   children die from meningococcal meningitis. I

15 have

16   seen children lose their limbs from

17 meningococcal

18   meningitis. I have seen children who have

19 become

20   mentally retarded from meningococcal meningitis.

21 Why

1   not prevent those terrible side effects and take

2 the

3   chance on the relapse and treat the relapse.

4   And the same is true for -- for

5 chickenpox.

6   We now have a vaccine for chickenpox. Why go

7 through

8   this anxiety about the child getting chickenpox?

9 And

10   the same for Haemophilus meningitis and

11 streptococcal

12   pneumonia, peritonitis, all of -- and meningitis

13 or

14   pneumonia. Why not give the vaccine and try to

15 prevent

16   these catastrophic -- potentially catastrophic

17   conditions?

18   And so what I -- what I plead for in

19 this

20   whole problem of looking after people with

21 chronic

1   disease is a kind of balance, weighing one thing

2   against the other, all the time looking for the

3 balance

4   so that the child or the adult can have a decent

5   quality of life.

6   Thank you very much.

7   (Video clip was stopped.)

8   SPECIAL MASTER MILLMAN: Mr. McHugh,

9 can you

10   tell me what the date of this lecture was?

11   MR. McHUGH: It appears to be 2010.

12   SPECIAL MASTER MILLMAN: Is there a

13 month in

14   2010?

15   MR. MILES: I would have to contact

16 NephCure

17   and get an exact date.

1   SPECIAL MASTER MILLMAN: That's all

2 right.

3   We'll just say 2010.

4   So do you think this might be Exhibit

5 102?

6   MR. McHUGH: It would probably be 10 -

7 - 110.

8   SPECIAL MASTER MILLMAN: 110?

9   MR. McHUGH: I'll make it 110.

10   SPECIAL MASTER MILLMAN: Okay. I

11 forget how

12   long I -- we had as 101 the components of the

13 flu

14   vaccines that you didn't bring because you

15 couldn't

16   print it out. So that's 101. Then you got

17 what, six

18   articles?

19   MR. McHUGH: Six articles.

20   SPECIAL MASTER MILLMAN: So that's

21 107.

1   So why isn't this 108?

2   MR. McHUGH: We can do that.

3   SPECIAL MASTER MILLMAN: Don't you

4 think?

5   MR. McHUGH: We can do that.

6   SPECIAL MASTER MILLMAN: Okay. 108,

7 and it's

8   2010.

9   THE WITNESS: Special Master, may I

10 say

11   something?

12   SPECIAL MASTER MILLMAN: One moment.

13   What is on my screen now? There's

14 something

15   else. Is this a transcript? This is a

16 transcript.

17   MR. McHUGH: No, that's -- that's not

18 an

1   official transcript. So we'll take that off.

2   MR. MILES: It's a script that I --

3   SPECIAL MASTER MILLMAN: I can't hear

4   you.

5   MR. MILES: I'm sorry. It's a script

6   that

7   I -- I created from the video.

8   SPECIAL MASTER MILLMAN: Oh, so you're

9   not

10 submitting that in evidence?

11   MR. McHUGH: I won't submit that. I

12 will

13 submit the video.

14   SPECIAL MASTER MILLMAN: Okay.

15   Now, sure, you can say whatever you

16 like.

17 But Mr. McHugh has -- obviously has the

18 opportunity to

19 ask you questions. Yes, Dr. Kaplan.

20   THE WITNESS: I shall wait for -- for

21 Mr. McHugh to ask the questions.

1   SPECIAL MASTER MILLMAN: I'm sorry?

2   THE WITNESS: I'll wait for the

3 question.

4   SPECIAL MASTER MILLMAN: Oh, yes.

5 What's

6   your question?

7   BY MR. McHUGH:

8   Q.   So yesterday, Dr. Quan, basically said

9 the

10   same thing, that he agrees that they should be

11   vaccinated because getting the disease is far

12 more

13   dangerous and --

14   SPECIAL MASTER MILLMAN: Hang on a

15 second.

1   Let's focus. Okay? In law school you learn to

2   focus

3   on issues. If you don't focus on the issues,

4   you fail

5   the test. In fact, you even fail the bar exam.

6   It is

7   not an issue before me whether or not JM should

8   have been immunized. The issue before me is

9   whether

10   the vaccination caused him to have significant

11   aggravation of his preexisting nephrotic

12   syndrome.

13   So asking the doctor, Is it a good

14   idea to

15   vaccinate or not, is irrelevant to me.

16   MR. McHUGH: Irrelevant to you. Okay.

17   BY MR. McHUGH:

18   Q.   Okay. But in this -- in this

19   particular

20   video, you do cite to a gentleman in England who

21   did do

1   a test and did see an increase in nephrotic

2 syndrome

3   after a vaccine; is that correct?

4   A.   The short answer is he did -- they

5 did.   The

6   longer answer is that that study was repeated in

7   another group of centers in London, in England,

8 by

9   Taylor, et al., and they did not show the same

10 results.

11   And if I may, that study was published

12 in

13   2003, and this was not in 2010 because a great

14 deal has

15   happened since 2010.   This NephCure Foundation

16 which I

17   helped to start actually was around 2004, and

18 that

19   paper from London, from Great Ormond Street had

20 just

21   come out in 2003.   And I was writing that paper

1 and had

1   not at that time seen Taylor's paper which came

2   out

3   subsequently.

4   And if I may, Special Master, I didn't

5   go

6   into this today because Dr. Quan in his -- one

7   of his

8   rebuttal letters to me actually backtracked on

9   this

10 particular study and added in Taylor's study,

11 because I

12 had brought Taylor's study to his attention.

13 And then

14 he said, Well, it's a little bit -- you know,

15 it's not

16 certain. We don't know the answer. So I think

17 the

18 answer to your question is a little bit longer

19 than

20 just saying yes or no.

21   Q.   Okay. But is it correct from all I've

1 been

2 hearing here that we don't know a lot of the

3 answers

4 with regard to nephrotic syndrome?

5   A.   I'm not sure where that question's

6 going

7 because we know a great deal about the nephrotic

8 syndrome. I spent this morning talking about

9 the

10 podocytes, about its structure, about its

11 function,

12 about the -- the genes that have been mutated,

13 about

14 the different -- about the different factors

15 that can

16 be involved, about the fact that the tyrosine

17 kinase

18 inhibitors can cause nephrotic syndrome. I

19 forgot to

20 mention that nonsteroidal and anti-inflammatory

21 agents,

1   like ibuprofen or intermedicine have been

2 associated as

3   causative agents of nephrotic syndrome.   I think

4 we

1   know a great deal.

2   We don't know everything because in

3   biology,

4   in medicine, we human beings don't know

5   everything

6   about any disease that you want to talk about.

7   We --

8   there are still unknowns. So yes, in nephrotic

9   syndrome, there are lots of unknowns, but we

10 know a

11 great deal.

12   Q.   Now, would you agree that after the

13 October 2nd flu shot, JM did not go into full

14 remission at all until after his stroke?

15   SPECIAL MASTER MILLMAN: October 1st?

16   MR. McHUGH: October 1st of 2009.

17   SPECIAL MASTER MILLMAN: Right.   I

18 think -- I

19 think I heard you say October 2nd.

20   MR. WISHARD: He said October 2nd.

21   MR. McHUGH: I did? Oh, October --

1   SPECIAL MASTER MILLMAN: He was

2 vaccinated

3   October 1st, 2009.

4   MR. McHUGH: Okay.   So let's say

5 October 2nd

6   is where --

7   SPECIAL MASTER MILLMAN: I'm sorry.

8 I'm a

9   little confused.

10   MR. McHUGH: October 2nd is when the

11 protein

12   went up.

13   SPECIAL MASTER MILLMAN: Right.   And

14 what do

574

1   you want to know? I've forgotten already what

2 your

3   question is.

4 BY MR. McHUGH:

5   Q.   Would you agree that -- that JM did

6 not

7   go into remission at any time after the

8 vaccination and

9   after the -- the October 2, 2009, increase in

10   proteinuria until after the stroke?

11   A.   I don't really understand that

12 question,

13 because my recollection is that, in fact, he was

14 taken

15   off the -- the Prograf because he was in

16 remission.

17 And they would not have taken him off the

18 Prograf were

19   he not in remission.

20   Q.   Okay.

21   SPECIAL MASTER MILLMAN: Doctor -- I'm

1 sorry.

2 Finish your answer.

3 THE WITNESS: So my answer to you,

4 sir, is

5 that I disagree with the premise of that

6 question.

7 SPECIAL MASTER MILLMAN: I don't

8 recall if

9 Dr. Quan said this, but I'm pretty sure Dr.

10 Bellanti

11 said it. In any event, I know I've heard, or

12 I've read

13 it, in the prehearing brief by Mr. McHugh, which

14 is:

15 Petitioner's view is -- and of course you --

16 you're an

17 expert nephrologist, pediatric nephrologist, and

18 you

19 should give your opinion because all of us are

20 not

21 doctors except the ones who are doctors.

1   But their view is that after the

2 October 1st,

3   2009, flu vaccination, JM never went into

4   remission. He -- it was always an unbeatable,

5   untreatable minimal change nephrotic syndrome

6 which had

7   kind of like that tide or wave image I presented

8   earlier before lunch. He would get better, he

9 would

10 get worse, but he never went into remission

11 again.

12   And you can disagree with that, but

13 that, I

14 take it -- and it may have been what Dr.

15 Bellanti said,

16 but I certainly picked that up from someplace in

17 the

18 petitioner's side. So I'm taking it that you

19 disagree,

20 Dr. Kaplan, with that characterization of JM's

21 course after October 1st, 2009.

1   THE WITNESS: Yes, Special Master.

2   SPECIAL MASTER MILLMAN: And how would

3 you

4   interpret his course after October 1st, 2009?

5   THE WITNESS: He -- he did not have a

6   completely smooth course. His course was not

7 smooth

8   because he did have what I called relapses where

9   Dr. Quan did not characterize his relapses.

10 What I

11   said earlier was blips in his protein or

12 breakthroughs.

13   But in my notes of -- here on page 3 of -- of

14   Exhibit A, the -- where I have the heading

15 "First

16   Relapse" at the bottom of that paragraph, I've

17 written

18   the -- that he sustained a prolonged remission

19 of

1   11 months while on Prograf. And then in June of

2   2011,

3   his parents asked Dr. Quan to stop the Prograf,

4   a

5   relapse occurred gradually by the end of July

6   2011, and

7   the nephrotic syndrome didn't respond to

8   Prednisone.

9   And then he had the -- the cerebral vascular

10 accident,

11 and then he did respond to Prednisone.

12   So I -- I don't -- I don't really

13 follow

14 the -- the question the way that you've asked

15 the

16 question.

17   SPECIAL MASTER MILLMAN: Okay. I

18 think what

19 you're saying is you don't agree with the

20 interpretation.

21   THE WITNESS: I'm sorry, ma'am, yes.

1   SPECIAL MASTER MILLMAN: You count in

2 this

3   Exhibit A which is your first --

4   THE WITNESS: Yes, ma'am.

5   SPECIAL MASTER MILLMAN: -- report,

6 that the

7   first relapse occurred obviously before the

8   vaccination. The second relapse occurred --

9 we're

10   talking about the October 1st, 2009,

11 vaccination. You

12   count a third relapse when Prednisone was being

13 weaned

14   in December of 2009; a fourth relapse in March

15 of 2010

16   when Prednisone was being tapered, and then he

17 was put

18   back on it; a fifth relapse on May 9th, 2010;

19 and then,

20   he had a prolonged remission of 11 months while

21 on

1   Prograf; and the sixth relapse after he was

2   taken off

3   in June 2011.

4   Is that correct?

5   THE WITNESS: Yes, ma'am.

6   SPECIAL MASTER MILLMAN: All right.

7   Go

8   ahead, Mr. McHugh.

9   BY MR. McHUGH:

10   Q.   Be fair to characterize Relapses 2

11 through 5

12 just that he could not be weaned off of the

13 steroids?

14   A.   That would be one way of

15 characterizing it.

16   Q.   And is it true that we're still

17 treating

18 nephrotic syndrome with -- with steroids?

19   A.   His nephrotic syndrome or in general?

20   Q.   In general.

21   A.   Yes, it's our first-line treatment.

1   Q.   Okay.

2   SPECIAL MASTER MILLMAN: Is minimal

3 change

4   nephrotic syndrome being treated with steroids?

5   THE WITNESS: Yes.   I understood Mr.

6 McHugh

7   to be referring to minimal change nephrotic

8 syndrome,

9   yes.

10   SPECIAL MASTER MILLMAN: Okay.

11   MR. McHUGH: I will continue to --

12   SPECIAL MASTER MILLMAN: When I hear

13 "in

14   general," I think, oh, we're from Alfred or

15 Alport or

1   whatever the heck it is, and it's all out there,

2   including adults. So you have to be specific.

3   THE WITNESS: Yes, ma'am.

4   SPECIAL MASTER MILLMAN: Even if Mr.

5   McHugh

6   is not specific, you have to be specific.

7   BY MR. McHUGH:

8   Q.   And is it true in most cases, the --

9   the

10   steroid work -- in most cases of nephrotic

11   syndrome,

12   the steroid does work and brings the thing under

13   control relatively quickly?

14   A.   That is correct.

15   Q.   Okay. Is it true that steroids are an

16   immune

17   suppressant drug?

18   A.   I'm not sure about how to answer that

19   question. They are anti-inflammatory. That is

20   the

21   case. But do they have effects on the immune

1 system

2 per se? That's -- that's more problematical.

3 But they

4 have been so characterized.

5   SPECIAL MASTER MILLMAN: Is

6 inflammation

7 unrelated to immune system?

8   THE WITNESS: So -- so they are

9 related to

10 each other, but there are different -- they're

11 different components of the immune system. So

12 yes,

13 I -- I would say they are characterized as anti

14 -- as

15 immunosuppressants, yes.

1   SPECIAL MASTER MILLMAN: If minimal

2 change

3   nephrotic syndrome is a podocytopathy and not an

4   immune-mediated illness, why, then, would a drug

5 like

6   Prednisone affect the course of the disease

7 since that

8   is anti-inflammatory?

9   THE WITNESS: Well, this -- this

10 question had

11   no clear answer for the longest time.   We were

12 using

13   Prednisone without having the faintest idea what

14 it

15   was -- what its pathways were, what it was doing

16 in

17   terms of minimal change nephrotic syndrome,

18 until this

19   paper that appeared about two years ago which

20 I've

21   referred to Clemens paper.   It appeared in

1 Nature, and

2   they suggested that the steroids were having an

3 effect

4   on the podocytes and the basement membrane

5 through this

6   Angio-Proteomie 4 chemical which has nothing to

7 do with

8   the immunological factors.

9   And -- and so this is still an

10 evolving

11   subject where people are now trying to

12 understand how

13   these agents are working by focusing on the cell

14 that's

15   injured in this condition, i.e., the podocytes

16 rather

17   than looking at other cells in the body.

18   SPECIAL MASTER MILLMAN: Go ahead,

19   Mr. McHugh.

20   BY MR. McHUGH:

21   Q.   When Dr. Quan states that he believes

1 that

1   the steroid is used because it does control the

2   immune

3   system, he is wrong?

4   A.   That is Dr. Quan's opinion. He's not

5   here to

6   discuss it with me. I cannot ask him what his

7   understanding is about the more recent studies.

8 So if

9   Dr. Quan has that opinion, that's fine. I would

10   venture to say that a lot of nephrologists still

11   believe that. And I'm not going to say that

12 he's

13   wrong.

14   But at the risk of being repetitious,

15 I would

16   say that it's an evolving subject, and that it

17 may turn

18   out that he is wrong in terms of nephrotic

19 syndrome.

20   Q.   So this is an area that is unsettled,

21 and

1   various experts have different opinions?

2   A.   If we are going to define an expert as

3   somebody who's actually done research in the

4 area,

5   somebody who has studied nephrotic syndrome,

6 compared

7   to somebody who has taken care of patients, then

8 we

9   have a difference of opinion as to who is an

10 expert.

11   So, for example, I look after -- I did

12 look

13   after patients with hypertension, but I did not

14   consider myself to be an expert in the

15 complicated

16   field of hypertension. I did look after

17 patients with

18   hemolytic uremic syndrome, and I did consider

19 myself to

20   be an expert because I had done so many studies

21 and

1   written so many papers on the subject.

2   When I reviewed Dr. Quan's publication

3   record, and he himself said he had not written

4 about

5   nephrotic syndrome or studied nephrotic

6 syndrome, so I

7   don't want to put myself up against Dr. Quan.

8 That's

9   not fair. I respect him, but that's his

10 opinion. If

11   you're talking about experts, we can start

12 pulling

13   arts, papers by Glassock, for example. I have

14 quoted

15   Glassock's paper. Glassock was one of the

16 preeminent

17   nephrologists in the world until he died

18 recently, and

19   he had spent a career studying nephrotic

20 syndrome.

21   Dr. Levinson may speak about him. And he had

1 shifted

2   completely away from the immune pathogenesis of

3   nephrotic syndrome to other theories, the ones

4 that

5   I've been talking about.

6   If we're going to talk about Dr.

7 William

8   Couser, who had -- was also a world expert on

9 nephrotic

10   syndrome, he does not mention minimal change

11 nephrotic

12   syndrome as an immune-mediated condition in the

13 paper

14   that I submitted which reviews the whole subject

15 of

16   nephrotic syndrome. I had said before that he

17 did

18   consider his own condition that he studied the

19   membranous gene in the immune mediated but not

20 the

21   minimal change.

1   Q.   Is it still believed that nephrotic

2 syndrome

1   follows in many cases a viral attack?

2   A.   There are patients who definitely do

3 have a

4   viral infection documented and develop nephrotic

5   syndrome. This was not the case with JM. There

6   is no documentation that he ever had a virus

7 infection.

8   So I do have to add that rider.

9   Q.   Now, you indicated that from a -- a

10   thrombosis in the artery of a young child was

11 very

12   rare; is that correct?

13   A.   What I had said specifically was that

14   cerebral vascular accidents, a thrombus in the

15 cerebral

16   artery of a child with nephrotic syndrome was

17 extremely

18   rare. I had elaborated afterwards by saying, in

19   response to the special master's question, that

20 this

21   occurs not infrequently in children with sickle

1 cell

2   disease, in children with vascular disorders.

3 But in

4   specifically minimal change nephrotic syndrome,

5 I had

6   said, yes, that is very rare. I'm trying to be

7   specific in terms of answering my question.

8   Q.   But it's -- it's very rare, but it

9 isn't

10   impossible.

11   SPECIAL MASTER MILLMAN: Did you say

12   "impossible"?

13   MR. McHUGH: Yes.

14   SPECIAL MASTER MILLMAN: We don't deal

15 with

1   possible and impossible here.

2   BY MR. McHUGH:

3   Q.   It is -- it is rare, but it does

4 happen?

5   A.   It is rare, but it has been

6 occasionally

7   reported.

8   MR. McHUGH: Nothing further, Your

9 Honor.

10   SPECIAL MASTER MILLMAN: That's it?

11 Thank

12   you.

13   Mr. Wishard, any redirect?

14   MR. WISHARD: Just for housekeeping

15 purposes,

16   he talked about three articles.   I just want to

17   identify for the record the three articles.

18   SPECIAL MASTER MILLMAN: Sure.   Go

19 ahead.

20   MR. WISHARD: Clement's is at Exhibit

21 C,

1   Tab 16.   Couser is at Exhibit O, and Glassock is

2 at

3   Exhibit C, Tab 14, just for the record because -

4 -

5   SPECIAL MASTER MILLMAN: Thank you.

6   MR. WISHARD: Beyond that, I have no

7 further

8   questions.

9   SPECIAL MASTER MILLMAN: All right.

10 Thank

11   you very much, Doctor.   I appreciate your

12 testimony.

13   THE WITNESS: Thank you, Special

14 Master.

15   SPECIAL MASTER MILLMAN: Is it Ms.

16 Soanes

17   who's up next?

18   MR. WISHARD: No. I am.

1   SPECIAL MASTER MILLMAN: You are. So

2 sorry.

3 Yes, Mr. Wishard would you like to call your

4 next

5 witness, please.

6   MR. WISHARD: Yes, please.

7   SPECIAL MASTER MILLMAN: Would you

8 like to

9 raise your right hand, please.

10 Thereupon--

11   ARNOLD LEVINSON, M.D.,

12 was called as a witness, and having been first

13 duly

14 sworn, was examined and testified as follows:

15

16   THE WITNESS: I do.

17   SPECIAL MASTER MILLMAN: Would you

18 state your

19 name and professional address for the record,

20 please.

21   THE WITNESS: My name is Arnold

1 Levinson. My

2   address is Radnor, Pennsylvania.

3   SPECIAL MASTER MILLMAN: Thank you

4 very much.

5   Your witness, Mr. Wishard.

6   MR. WISHARD: Thank you, ma'am.

7

8   DIRECT EXAMINATION

9   BY MR. WISHARD:

10   Q.   You were asked your professional

11 address.

12   A.   Oh.

13   Q.   What is -- no, that's fine.

1   What is your current profession?

2   A.   My professional is -- title is

3 Emeritus

4 Professor of Medicine and Neurology at the

5 University

6 of Pennsylvania, now called Perelman School of

7 Medicine.

8   Q.   Okay.

9   SPECIAL MASTER MILLMAN: Okay.   Why

10 did I

11 think you were an immunologist for some reason?

12   THE WITNESS: Why did you think what?

13   SPECIAL MASTER MILLMAN: You're not an

14 immunologist.

15   THE WITNESS: I am an immunologist.

16   SPECIAL MASTER MILLMAN: But you're a

17 professor of medicine and neurology?

18   THE WITNESS: And neurology.   I'm an

19 immunologist in the department of medicine and a

20 secondary appointment in neurology because I

21 have

1 studied neuroimmunology during the course of my

2 37 years or so at the University of

3 Pennsylvania.

4   SPECIAL MASTER MILLMAN: Thank you

5 very much.

6   Go ahead, Mr. Wishard.

7   MR. WISHARD: Thank you.

8 BY MR. WISHARD:

9   Q. Are you now retired?

10   A. I am now retired. You're going to

11 have to

1   speak up because I'm -- I've only got one

2 hearing aid

3   in today.

4   Q.   I will do that. Okay.

5   A.   Okay. Thank you.

6   Q.   If I have to lean forward, I don't

7 want to --

8   SPECIAL MASTER MILLMAN: No. We

9 project.

10   This is what we do. See, lungs, project.

11   BY MR. WISHARD:

12   Q.   When did you retire from practice?

13   A.   I retired approximately three years

14 ago.

15   Q.   Okay. When -- can you tell the

16 special

17   master a little bit about your educational

18 background?

19   A.   Sure. I'll start with medical school.

20 I

21   graduated from the University of Maryland

1 Medical

2   School in 1969. I then did a medicine residency

3 at

4   what is now called Bayview Johns Hopkins. I

5 completed

6   that, and then I decided I wanted to become an

7   immunologist and had no research training.

8   So I was fortunate to get a position

9 at the

10   University of Pennsylvania where I spent a year

11 getting

12   immersed in basic immunology, then went out to

13 the

14   University of California in San Francisco. The

15 name of

16   Robert Good was mentioned earlier today. I

17 worked with

18   a fellow by the name of Hugh Fudenberg who was

19 also

20   considered to be a father of clinical

21 immunology. And

1   I spent a year there, came back for two years of

2   postdoctoral fellowship in clinical immunology

3 and

4   allergy at the University of Pennsylvania School

5 of

6   Medicine. And then did my Army service at the

7 Walter

8   Reed Army Medical Center where I ran the

9 clinical

10   immunology laboratory. Came back to Penn in

11 1978 and

12   stayed there until essentially 2014.

13   During my time there, I spent a year

14 at the

15   University of Oxford in Sir William Dunn school

16   learning molecular immunology.

17   SPECIAL MASTER MILLMAN: Thank you.

18 BY MR. WISHARD:

19   Q.   Do you hold board certifications?

20   A.   Yes. I'm board certified in internal

21 medicine and allergy and immunology.

1   Q.   When you -- before you retired from

2   Penn, did

3   you have any teaching responsibilities?

4   A.   I had a lot of teaching

5   responsibilities. I

6   lectured to medical students and immunology

7   graduate

8   students and, in addition, I was responsible for

9   supervising interns, residents on ward medicine

10 team

11 and, also, allergy and immunology fellows,

12 postdoctoral

13 fellows.

14   Q.   Did you hold any -- I understand, I

15 think you

16 were an associate dean at one point in time of

1   research; is that correct?

2   A.   Well, in terms of my tenure at Penn, I

3 worked

4   myself through the ranks up to professor of

5 medicine

6   and neurology. In addition, I held the position

7 of

8   chief or chair of the Penn Center for Clinical

9   Immunology. I was the chair of the allergy and

10   immunology department as well as its training

11 program

12   director. And then ultimately stepped down from

13 those

14   positions to become an associate dean for

15 research in

16   the medical school.

17   Thank you for reminding me of that.

18   Q.   When you taught, who did you teach,

19 medical

20   students, residents, fellows, all of the above?

21   A.   All of the above.

1   Q.   Okay.   And when you taught, what did

2 you

3   mostly teach on?

4   A.   Well, I taught primarily on what we

5 now call

6   clinical immunology.   And that was really

7 translating

8   basic immunology into clinical medicine,

9 particularly

10   as it related to hypersensitivity disorders,

11 including

12   autoimmune diseases and allergic diseases, IGE-

13 mediated

14   allergic diseases.   But all kinds of

15 hypersensitivity

16   diseases and immune deficiency.

17   Q.   In addition to teaching, did you also

18 conduct

19   research on autoimmune issues?

1   A.   Yes, I conducted research on

2 autoimmunity

3   issues, fair to say.

4   Q.   And you published your research?

5   A.   Yes, I did.

6   Q.   And have you also worked in the --

7 working on

8   book chapters or books in terms of autoimmunity

9 and

10   immunity?

11   A.   Yes.

12   Q.   How about in any type of medical

13 journals?

14   A.   Yes. Obviously -- not obviously, but

15 I

16   published several papers along the way that

17 related to

18   my research interests, particularly as they

19 pertained

20   to autoimmunity, but more of an overview as they

21   pertain to adaptive immune mechanisms,

1 particularly

2   T cells and B cells, particularly as those

3 mechanisms

4   related to autoimmune disease. And along the

5 way was

6   interested in mechanism of -- mechanisms of

7 immunologic

8   tolerance and breach of immunologic tolerance

9 that led

10   to or leads to autoimmune disease, particularly

11 with

12   regard to a neuroimmunologic disease called

13 myasthenia

14   gravis.

15   Q. Now, your CV has been made part of the

16 record

17   as Exhibit E. And on your CV at that time, the

18 last

19   publication was in 2013.

20   Have you had any additional

21 publications

1   since 2013 that have been published?

2   A.   Yes.   I'm surprised you don't have

3 that.

4   There are two papers that relate to

5 hypersensitivity

6   responses that were made by patients in response

7 to a

8   new type of treatment that served -- that was

9 hoped it

10   would serve, the treatment would serve as an

11   anticoagulant.   The treatment is referred to as

12 an

13   aptamer, which is an oligonucleotide that

14 combined to a

15   protein and knock out the protein.   In this

16 case, the

17   idea was to knock out an anticoagulant.   I was

18 involved

19   in those studies and, in particular, the senior

20 author

21   on a paper that examined allergic reactions to

1 that

2   molecule.

3   Q.   Have you served as reviewer on any

4   peer-reviewed journals?

5   A.   Yes.

6   Q.   Just name a few.

7   A.   Journal of Allergy and Clinical

8 Immunology,

9   Clinical Immunology, Journal of Neurologic

10 Science,

11   Journal of Clinical Investigation, Lancet, et

12 cetera,

13   et cetera.

14   Q.   And in terms of your practice, during

15 the

16   course of your practice and your research have

17 you

18   received any honors or awards?

19   A.   Yes. I -- during the course of my

20 practice,

1   I was -- received the moniker of "top doc" in

2 allergy

3   and immunology and -- in Philadelphia, and also

4   whatever that thing is called, American's top

5 doctors

6   over a period of a number of years.

7   In the teaching arena, I received

8 three

9   teaching awards over my tenure at Penn, one of

10 which --

11   I'm proud of all of them, but one of which I'm

12   particularly proud of is called the Leonard

13 Berwick

14   Award, which is an award given to an individual

15 in the

16   medical school who is recognized for bridging

17 basic

18   science and clinical medicine. In addition, I

19 was

20   elected to American Society for Clinical

21 Investigation

1   which recognizes individuals who have shown --

2   M.D.s

3   who have shown expertise in clinical

4   investigation as

5   physicians, scientists in particular. I was

6   elected

7   president of the Clinical Immunologists Society;

8   chair

9   of the American Board of Allergy and Immunology,

10   the

11   certifying board for people who are going to go

12   in to

13   be certified in allergy and immunology; and also

14   elected to the board of directors of the

15   American -- of

16   the clinical and allergy by a group by American

17   Association of Allergy and Immunologists where I

18   was

19   then internally elected as the chair of the

20   research

21   and training division.

1   Q.   Have you lectured on the immunology

2 and

1   clinical immunology issues?

2   A.   Yes.

3   MR. WISHARD: Special Master, I would

4 offer

5   Dr. Levinson as an expert in immunology and

6 clinical

7   immunology.

8   SPECIAL MASTER MILLMAN: Thank you.

9   Mr. McHugh?

10   MR. McHUGH: No objection.

11   SPECIAL MASTER MILLMAN: Thank you.

12 You are

13   so admitted.

14   MR. WISHARD: Thank you.

15   BY MR. WISHARD:

16   Q.   Dr. Levinson, you have been asked --

17 you were

18   asked to review this case starting several years

19 ago,

20   actually, when your first reports were produced.

21   Did you have an opportunity during the

1 course

2 of your work on this case to review all the

3 exhibits

4 that were filed by petitioner including the

5 medical

6 records, the expert reports, and the medical

7 literature?

8   A.   Well, all of those except the ones

9 that were

10 filed this weekend or whenever it was.

11   Q.   Except for the most recent ones, which

12 we'll

13 talk about in a second.

14   And did you -- you were obviously

15 present for

1   the testimony of Dr. Quan, Dr. Bellanti, and

2   Mr. Miles --

3   A.   Yes, I was.

4   Q.   -- correct?

5   Have you reached an opinion on if the

6   October 1st, 2009, flu vaccine significantly

7 aggravated

8   JM's minimal change disease?

9   A.   Yes, I reached an opinion which hasn't

10 been

11   changed since I have been in this courtroom.

12   Q.   Okay. And just for the record, you

13 authored

14   two reports which, for the record, are Exhibit D

15 and

16   Exhibit J.

17   And based upon your review of

18 everything, do

19   you believe to a more likely than not standard

20 that the

21   flu vaccine on October 1st, 2009, significantly

1   aggravated JM's nephrotic syndrome, which is

2   minimal change disease in this case?

3   A.   No, I do not believe that that

4 vaccination on

5   October 1st either led to a relapse or

6 exacerbated a

7   relapse.

8   Q.   Okay. And do you also hold that same

9 opinion

10   in terms of whether or not the October 1st,

11 2009, flu

12   vaccine, it was in any way -- by receiving it,

13 that it

14   in any way exacerbated or caused JM to suffer

15 from

16   a CVA 22 months later?

1   A.   Yes, I have a strong opinion that that

2 vaccination did not lead to the CVA.

3   Q.   And I'm asking your opinions to a more

4 likely

5 than not standard.

6   A.   That -- that more likely than not, it

7 did not

8 lead to the CVAs.

9   Q.   Now, you were here for Dr. Kaplan's

10 testimony

11 this morning summarizing his thoughts on -- as -

12 - as a

13 pediatric nephrologist regarding the facts of

14 JM's

15 case.

16   Do you have anything to add to that?

17 Otherwise I'm going to focus on the immunology.

18   A.   No.

19   Q.   Okay. And anything to add or your

20 view might

21 be slightly different than anything that Dr.

1 Kaplan

2   said on the immunology issues this morning?

3   A.   Well, I think he said one thing that I

4 -- I

5   do differ in my opinion, and that is in response

6 to a

7   question he mentioned that in cases of

8   post-streptococcal glomerular nephritis an

9 anamnestic

10   response might occur. And I agree with that

11 point.

12   But as a spinoff of that, I think a

13 message

14   that came out was that an anamnestic response

15 might be

16   responsible for what happened with regard to the

17   development of the nephrotic syndrome in JM.

18 And

1   just in case that that's what was discussed, and

2 I may

3   have heard it wrong, but I -- I strongly

4 disagree with

5   that.

6   Q.   Okay. And we'll get into an

7 anamnestic

8   response and your views on that in a moment when

9 we go

10   through the immunology issues in the case.

11   You would agree that -- with the

12 diagnosis

13   that JM has nephrotic syndrome minimal change

14   disease?

15   A.   Yes.

16   Q.   And you would also agree that he had

17 an

18   elevation in his protein -- of his protein

19 levels

20   within 24 hours of receiving the flu vaccine on

21   October 1st, 2009?

1   A.   Yes.

2   Q.   Now, I want to talk to you a little

3 bit about

4   the theory, theories that have been proposed

5 here or

6   raised through the testimony of Dr. Bellanti

7 mostly,

8   although Dr. Quan did talk a little bit about it

9 as

10   well, with the components being the innate

11 immune

12   system and the adaptive immune system.

13   A.   Right.

14   Q.   The hypothesis that's been proposed by

15   petitioners here, do you agree with it?

16   A.   No.

1   Q.   And let's first start with -- perhaps

2 we

3   should start with the adaptive immune system.

4   A.   That's fine.

5   Q.   In terms of your understanding and

6 your

7   expertise in the adaptive immune system, why in

8 this

9   case does the hypothesis or the theory proposed

10 by

11   Dr. Bellanti not work for JM?

12   A.   So let -- before I address that

13 specific, let

14   me just say that my understanding of what Dr.

15 Bellanti

16   is proposing, at least now, that's changed a bit

17 from

18   what he proposed before, but the latest

19 iteration has

20   two pillars, one being that there's an innate

21 immune

1   component that he thinks accounts for the rather

2 brisk

3   development of the proteinuria following the

4   vaccination. And then a second pillar or second

5   component, that of an adaptive immune response

6 that

7   occurs later on, days to weeks, whatever, and I

8   heard -- I think I heard him say that that

9 accounts for

10   the chronicity or the relapses that occur in

11 this

12   disease, so ...

13   Q.   Post vaccination.

14   A.   Post vaccination, right. So let's

15 start with

16   the adaptive immune response.

17   SPECIAL MASTER MILLMAN: And I think

18 this

19   morning, 'cause we put him on -- I put him on

20 the stand

1   to answer whether the components of the 2008 and

2   2009

3   flu vaccinations are sufficiently similar to

4   support

5   his theory that there was an anamnestic response

6   to

7   explain the rapidity of what he considers to be

8   the --

9   the first sign of relapse which would be within

10   24 hours. And I think he said that not only

11 what you

12   just repeated from yesterday's testimony, but

13 that that

14   anamnestic response not only made the innate

15 immune

16   system respond quickly, which you would expect

17 anyway,

18   but made the adaptive immune system respond

19 quicker as

20   well.

21   THE WITNESS: Right. Okay. So let's

1 talk

2   about the adaptive immune response and what's

3 referred

4   to by the term "an anamnestic response,"

5   notwithstanding the fact that Dr. Bellanti made

6 a

7   schematic of that on his slide show.

8   When immunologists talk about an

9 anamnestic

10   response, they're talking about a specific

11 immune

12   response that occurs following an encounter with

13 an

14   antigen that that patient or that host had

15 encountered

16   or seen before. And when we talk about specific

17 immune

18   responses in an adaptive immune response, we're

19 talking

20   about T cell responses and B cell responses,

21 that are

1   antigen specific.

2   And we know, as Dr. Bellanti showed in

3 his

1   schematic, that the antibody responses in a

2 primary

3   immune response that occur the first time a

4 patient

5   sees an antigen, occurs to the IGG responses at

6 least

7   during the period of sensitization, occur

8 anywhere from

9   10 to 21 days after the immunization or

10 encounter with

11   the antigen. The T cell effector type responses

12 that

13   occur, helper cytolytic, Dr. Bellanti referred

14 to them

15   as whatever, they occur a little bit later but

16 usually

17   within two weeks.

18   However, when an individual encounters

19 that

20   same antigen again, the response is indeed

21 telescoped.

1   It occurs over a much shorter period of time.

2 And when

3   I'm talking about the response, I'm talking

4 about the

5   specific antibody response and T cell response

6 to that

7   same antigen that's now encountered a second

8 time or

9   even a third time. So when does it typically

10 occur?

11   With regard to antibodies, at least,

12 that

13   response occurs anywhere from three to seven, a

14 few

15   days later. In regard to T cells, it usually

16 occurs

17   within -- depending upon the nature of the

18 response

19   that you're looking at, the organ that's

20 affected,

21   because when you're measuring antibodies, you're

1   measuring antibodies in the serum.   When you're

2 looking

3   at T cell response in vivo in the patient,

4 you're

5   looking at a response that affects some organ,

6 it

1   usually occurs within a few days to -- a few

2 days,

3   three, occasionally two, but three to five to

4 seven

5   days. Okay. Again, but remember, it depends

6 upon the

7   organ where you're looking.

8   So let's stop, sit back, take a

9 breath, and

10   think about what we've heard so far. What we've

11 been

12   talking about is a disease called MCD. It's

13 called MCD

14   for a specific reason, as you heard Dr. Kaplan

15 describe

16   eloquently. And that reason is they're --

17 there's no

18   inflammatory reaction. There is no evidence of

19 any

20   immunologic reactants that are -- can be seen,

21 can be

1   detected within the involved kidney. So in a

2 certain

3   respect, thinking about an anamnestic response

4 is moot

5   because we're not dealing with a specific

6   antigen-induced T cell response or antibody

7 response

8   that anybody knows about in this disease. All

9 right?

10   That's Point No. 1. That's an important point.

11 A

12   really important point because we're dealing

13 with

14   minimal change disease.

15   We're not dealing with membranous

16 nephropathy

17   which you heard, again, Dr. Kaplan talk about

18 today

19   where there is an antibody, an auto antibody,

20 that's

21   been described that reacts with a podocyte

1 antigen

2   called PLA2R. Now, that's a situation where if

3 there

4   was an encounter with an antigen, a foreign

5 antigen

1   that shared molecules, you know very well about

2   molecular mimicry, that it's possible that an

3 antibody

4   response or an adaptive immune response could be

5   important in the pathogenesis of that disease,

6 that

7   type of membranous nephropathy because an

8 antibody is

9   involved. And if the patient had encountered

10 the

11   antigen that that molecular mimics the cell

12 antigen,

13   PLA2R, had encountered that antigen before and

14 then saw

15   it a second or third time, there could be an

16 anamnestic

17   response. But that's not what we're dealing

18 with here

19   in minimal change disease.

20   So whether this vaccine that he got in

21 2009

1   shares epitopes or had some of the same

2 components as

3   were found in 2008 is moot. Because antibodies,

4 as

5   best as we can tell, or for that matter,

6   antigen-specific T cells are not involved in the

7   pathogenesis of this disease. That's an

8 important

9   point that I want to drive home so the Court

10   understands that, because there was a lot of

11 time spent

12   by Dr. Bellanti on anamnestic responses. I

13 pointed out

14   in my initial report or maybe it was my -- yeah,

15 my

16   initial report as well as my second report, that

17 it's

18   irrelevant to this case.

19   Again, if we're talking about a case

20 like

21   membranous nephropathy or post-streptococcal

1 glomerular

1   nephropathy where components of the adaptive

2 immune

3   system are involved in the pathogenesis, then it

4   becomes very important to talk about and think

5 about.

6   But not so in this case.

7   SPECIAL MASTER MILLMAN: You did not

8 mention

9   in your answer the innate immune system. And

10 that

11   Dr. Bellanti emphasized was also involved here

12 which

13   would explain the almost instantaneous

14 "reaction."

15   That is, sometime within a day of the

16 vaccination

17   October 1st, 2009, the innate immune system,

18 which I

19   tend to think of as allergy, but that that was

20 involved

21   and that also led to the adaptive immune system

1   functioning, carrying on the chronicity of this,

2 if

3   this was all one relapse.

4   Have you any opinion about the innate?

5   THE WITNESS: Sure. So Mr. Wishard

6 asked me

7   to start on adaptive immunity, which I did.

8   SPECIAL MASTER MILLMAN: That's right.

9 So

10 you know I jump in, so I jumped.

11   THE WITNESS: Well, whatever.

12 Whatever.

13   Yeah, so -- well, we've got --

14 petitioners

15 have a problem here. And the problem is that

16 the

17 proteinuria started probably around eight to ten

18 --

19 depending upon when he got the vaccine, but it

20 sounds

21 like he got the vaccine late in the day.

1   SPECIAL MASTER MILLMAN: 3:30 to 4:00

2 p.m.

3   THE WITNESS: Yeah, 4:00 o'clock.   So

4 we're

5   talking well less than 24 hours.   So they have a

6   problem in -- if indeed -- well, I'm sure they

7 do

8   believe that the vaccine was -- was the

9 provocator

10   here.   But they have a problem explaining that

11   immunologically.   So how could they possibly

12 explain

13   that in immunologic terms?

14   The only way they could explain it is,

15 well,

16   innate immunity occurs, as you heard, within a

17 period

18   of hours to, you know, 24 hours.   And, well,

19 maybe

20   that's what did it, and that's what they're

21 putting all

1   their eggs on.

2   Now, here's the problem: The problem

3 is

4   there's a giant leap of faith, as far as I'm

5 concerned,

6   from going from a needle with a vaccine injected

7 into

8   presumably the deltoid muscle, I'm guessing, but

9 maybe

10   it was elsewhere and the father can tell us, but

11 at any

12   rate, not injected into the kidney, injected

13 into a

14   remote tissue, probably muscle. How a vaccine

15 injected

16   into that muscle elicits an innate immune

17 response that

18   somehow winds up in the kidney, not only in the

19 kidney,

20   but in a very special compartment of the kidney

21 which

1   you've heard a great deal about, the epithelial

2   podocytes.

1   Now, I heard Dr. Bellanti say

2 yesterday, made

3   a statement that I think is totally unsupported.

4 And

5   that is, that, well, we know that vaccine -- flu

6   vaccine induces a tremendous cytokine response.

7 I have

8   no idea where he pulled that from. I'm not

9 aware of

10   any evidence. It's possible that he's actually

11   conflating what goes on with wild-type influenza

12   infection and flu vaccine. We know in terms of

13 a

14   wild-type influenza vaccine that infection, that

15 there

16   can be a tremendous kind of cytokine response.

17 And he

18   or somebody used the term "cytokine storm,"

19 which can

20   result in damage to most organs of the body.

21 That's a

1   very serious clinical syndrome. But it does

2 occur in

3   influenza infection and, in fact, that's what

4 most

5   people died from, that and pneumococcal

6 infection, in

7   the 1918 influenza outbreak. But there's

8 absolutely no

9   evidence that I'm aware of that influenza

10 vaccine, or

11   for that matter, any other vaccination, leads to

12 a

13   tremendous outpouring of cytokines.

14   So I have a lot of difficulty

15 processing the

16   notion that a flu vaccination leads to

17 tremendous

18   cytokine response that somehow damages the foot

19   processes of the podocyte.

20   SPECIAL MASTER MILLMAN: Of the

21 kidneys?

1   THE WITNESS: Of the kidney.

1   SPECIAL MASTER MILLMAN: Now, we had

2 some

3   discussion with Dr. Kaplan about that, and he

4 said it's

5   not this pattern of step by step.   The theories

6 that

7   I've heard in many other cases is that it's a

8 normal

9   thing for vaccines to produce cytokines because

10   cytokines induce the B cells to perform, to

11 create

12   antibodies, and the T cells to do whatever they

13 do.

14   THE WITNESS: Right.

15   SPECIAL MASTER MILLMAN: It's just

16 that

17   aberrant cytokines producing inflammation cause

18   whatever illness the petitioner's claiming.   And

19 so I

20   took that as what Dr. Bellanti was saying, that

21 this

1   cytokine abnormality affected the kidneys and

2   produced

3   in the first day the excess protein, the plus

4   three

5   proteinuria, that was registered for October

6   2nd, 2009.

7   THE WITNESS: Okay.

8   SPECIAL MASTER MILLMAN: I take it you

9   disagree.

10   THE WITNESS: Question?

11   MR. WISHARD: She said, Do you

12 disagree?

13   SPECIAL MASTER MILLMAN: In terms of

14 do you

15 agree or disagree?

16   THE WITNESS: Yeah, I disagree. And I

17 mean,

18 I agree with everything you said in terms of

19 what

20 you've learned during these proceedings. And

21 that is,

1   there is a -- an early cytokine response that's

2 a local

3   response. It occurs in the local draining lymph

4 node.

5   If he got the shot in his arm, then his axillary

6 nodes

7   where the antigen winds up because it's carried

8 there

9   by macrophages, induces a cytokine response.

10 But a

11   cytokine response that's not measured in terms

12 of

13   tremendous release of cytokines.

14   And the -- the corollary is, then, if

15 one

16   believes that, one has to explain how those

17 cytokines

18   actually damaged just the podocytes in -- in the

19 kidney

20   because JM just had MCD. And by the way, you've

21   heard this before, no other child has been

1 reported to

2 develop MCD, if I got the literature right and

3 heard

4 the testimony right, after a flu vaccine. All

5 right?

6 So -- but -- but let's come back to your point.

7   And so I don't agree with what Dr.

8 Bellanti

9 said.

10   SPECIAL MASTER MILLMAN: And you would

11 expect

12 to --

13   THE WITNESS: Oh, and can I say one

14 other

15 thing?

16   SPECIAL MASTER MILLMAN: Yes, of

17 course.

18   THE WITNESS: Let's make one other

19 point

20 which I think is as -- also almost as important

21 or

1   maybe as important as the whole anamnestic issue

2 which

1   has been talked about here. So let's step back

2   and

3   think about this.

4   We talked about the adaptive immune

5   system as

6   being the immune system that responds to

7   specific

8   antigens. And we talked about how an anamnestic

9   response occurs when that specific antigen is

10 encountered again; right? I mean, I think we

11 all have

12 that. And Dr. Bellanti talked about these

13 memory cells

14 that are already put out and ready to go to war

15 who get

16 recruited -- which get recruited after, in this

17 case,

18 an immunization. All right? And can cause a

19 booster

20 response to the immunizing antigen. So that --

21 there's

1   memory there; right?

2   Well, let's think about an innate

3 immune

4   response. If everybody's on the same page, an

5 innate

6   immune response has no memory. There's no

7 memory to an

8   innate immune response. We've heard about cells

9 like

10   macrophages, dendritic cells, neutrophils,

11 acidophils,

12   mass cells and so forth. So if an innate immune

13 cell

14   is going to respond to whatever the stimulant is

15 that

16   the host encounters, it will respond. It

17 doesn't need

18   to see that antigen or that foreign substance

19 more than

20   once. The response will not be increased if an

21 innate

1   immune cell sees like a macrophage, dendritic

2 cells,

3   what have you, that's part of the component of

4 the

1   immune system. It will not increase its

2 response the

3   second time around or the third time around.

4   So, again, let's take a step back and

5 think

6   about what's been proposed here. What's been

7 proposed

8   is that there's an -- an innate immune response

9 that's

10   responsible for the brisk development of

11 proteinuria in

12   JM. Well, gee, JM, as has been pointed out

13   by Mr. McHugh and Dr. Bellanti this morning, has

14   clearly seen the same vaccine before, except for

15 a

16   shift in one of the components.

17   So why didn't he make an innate immune

18   response before, if you accept the fact that you

19   don't -- from the standpoint of the innate

20 immune

21   system, you don't need to see the antigen?

1 What's

2 changed? You can make that argument for an

3 anamnestic

4 response. But I have already dispelled, I

5 think, I

6 hope, for everybody's understanding, the fact

7 that an

8 anamnestic response, even if he had one, to

9 influenza

10 antigen isn't relevant here.

11   SPECIAL MASTER MILLMAN: For the

12 innate

13 system.

14   THE WITNESS: For this case.

15   SPECIAL MASTER MILLMAN: For the

16 adaptive

17 system. Sorry.

18   THE WITNESS: For the adaptive system;

19 right.

1   SPECIAL MASTER MILLMAN: It's only

2 relevant

3   for the innate system.

4   THE WITNESS: It's only --

5   SPECIAL MASTER MILLMAN: The first

6 part of

7   that graph --

8   THE WITNESS: No, no, no, no.

9   SPECIAL MASTER MILLMAN: In this case

10 --

11   THE WITNESS: That's not an anamnestic

12   response. I'm sorry.

13   SPECIAL MASTER MILLMAN: What's not an

14   anamnestic response?

15   THE WITNESS: The little part of the

16 first

17   day or two days is not an -- that's not how we

18 describe

19   an anamnestic response.

20   SPECIAL MASTER MILLMAN: My only

21   understanding of an anamnestic response is

1 somebody

2 who's allergic to something, a bee sting,

3 peanuts, I

4 don't know what else is out there.

5   THE WITNESS: Okay.

6   SPECIAL MASTER MILLMAN: And you have

7 one bee

8 sting, you swell. You have a second bee sting,

9 you're

10 gasping. The third bee sting, you're dead.

11   THE WITNESS: Right. Got you. I need

12 to

13 help you with that one, with all --

14   SPECIAL MASTER MILLMAN: That's fine.

1   THE WITNESS: -- due respect. I heard

2 you

3   say that yesterday and I said, Uh-oh. So let me

4 try to

5   help you.

6   SPECIAL MASTER MILLMAN: Do help me.

7   THE WITNESS: Okay. So you heard

8   Dr. Bellanti say, and rightfully so, the immune

9 system

10   is very complex. There are multiple components

11 of the

12   immune system, as you've heard and as I have

13 said. You

14   also heard -- you might have heard him mention

15   yesterday an IGE antibody. And, in fact, when

16 you

17   described the innate immune response as being an

18   allergic response, he correctly corrected you.

19 He

20   said, well, most of us think about an allergic -

21 - an

1   allergic response, at least, in the pure sense,

2   as an

3   IGE-mediated mechanism.

4   Now, those IGE-mediated responses have

5   a

6   totally characteristic time course. They're

7   called

8   immediate hypersensitivity responses for a

9   reason

10 because they manifest within 10 to 15 minutes in

11 most

12 cases. So when you're referring to those

13 individuals

14 who develop anaphylaxis after -- because they're

15 allergic to bee venom or allergic to peanut

16 proteins,

17 they're developing a very particular type of

18 immune

19 response mechanism. Or at least they're

20 manifesting

21 it, and that's an IGE-type of response.

1   SPECIAL MASTER MILLMAN: And that's

2 not an

3   innate?

4   THE WITNESS: No, it's not innate.

5 It's an

6   adaptive immune response that is very different

7 than

8   the IGG or T cell mediated immune responses that

9 we're

10   generally talking about. That's not to say you

11   can't -- it's an immediate reaction. There is

12 no

13   evidence whatsoever, none, zero, nil, as you

14 heard that

15   term before today, that IGE antibodies, or for

16 that

17   matter, any flavor, any class of antibodies is

18 involved

19   in the pathogenesis of MCD.

20   So I hope I clarified that point --

21   SPECIAL MASTER MILLMAN: Thank you.

1   THE WITNESS: -- at least with regard

2 to that

3   very early type of -- you described. That's not

4 really

5   anamnestic response because they occur, boom.

6   SPECIAL MASTER MILLMAN: So what is

7 the

8   innate immune response?

9   THE WITNESS: Well, so what is the

10 innate

11   immune response? You heard about a number of

12 different

13   types of phagocytic cells, a number of different

14 types

15   of cells that respond in a nonspecific -- they

16 respond

17   quickly and in a relatively -- well, not

18 relatively,

19   but in an antigen nonspecific fashion. Some of

20 these

21   cells have receptors, but they bind to groups of

1   antigens. And you referred to, I think, some of

2 them

3   yesterday, these PAMPs and DAMPs, that you --

4 PAMPs are

5   molecular motifs that are expressed on classes

6 of

7   bacteria like endotoxin containing bacteria.

8 They

9   respond to DAMPs which are a damage associated

10 to

11   molecular motifs after tissues have been --

12 after

13   tissues have been damaged. They're components

14 of cells

15   that are called inflammasomes, not like

16 receptors which

17   when stimulated -- they all respond with a

18   relatively -- relatively quickly. Some of them

19 are

20   associated with the release of -- many of them

21 are

1   associated with the release of cytokines,

2 chemokines,

3   and what have you, as Dr. Bellanti talked about

4   yesterday.

5   SPECIAL MASTER MILLMAN: All right.

6 If you

7   could give me a scenario by timing of what you

8 expect

9   in this case when JM received a flu vaccination

10   3:30, 4:00 o'clock p.m. on October 1st, just

11 take me

12   through timewise and what's happening in the

13 response

14   that you would expect from receiving a flu

15 vaccination

16   and it's not his first.

17   THE WITNESS: Okay.   That's -- that's

18 fine.

19   Well, what I would expect is that the antigen

20 would be

21   trafficked, that it was deposited in his muscle

1   that's -- it was in his arm. It would be

2 deposited,

1   taken up by macrophages, dendritic cells and

2 carried

3   into the draining lymph node, probably in his

4 axilla.

5   There, the antigen peptides, the antigen would

6 have

7   been chewed up by what was referred to yesterday

8 as

9   antigen presenting cells into component bits

10 called

11   peptides of the protein in association with the

12 major

13   histocompatibility antigens on the surface of

14 those

15   antigen presenting cells to T cells. It also

16 would be

17   presented to B cells.

18   Now, remember that he -- he's seen the

19   antigen before, at least some of the antigens

20 before.

21   So there will be some T cells that are

1 trafficking

2 between the lymph and blood that arrive into the

3 area

4 that have been already out there. And as I

5 think was

6 said, newer antigens will be seen by smaller

7 numbers of

8 T cells and B cells, and those cells will

9 undergo a

10 series of activation events which are

11 characterized by

12 certain molecules that lead to what we refer to

13 as

14 signal transduction, you know. So the cells are

15 flooded with signals to do their thing.

16 Their thing starts off with some

17 proliferation. They differentiate as well as

18 differentiate to more mature effector cells,

19 cells that

20 are able to carry out effector function, kill.

21 If it's

1   cytotoxin, CDAT cells, kill whatever might be

2 out there

1   to be killed, help to -- if they're CD4 cells,

2   to help

3   B cells differentiate because B cells in many

4   cases or

5   in most cases depending upon the nature of the

6   antigen,

7   need help from the B cells -- from the T cells

8   to get

9   signals that will induce them to differentiate

10 all the

11 way to the point of becoming antibody secreting

12 plasma

13 cells.

14   And then the cells go -- traffic --

15 traffic

16 out into the periphery. In the case of T cells,

17 they'll ultimately traffic to the scene of the

18 crime,

19 wherever the antigen is because the antigens

20 there draw

21 the T cells into the combat zone and the T cells

1 do

2   their thing. B cells go to the spleen, go to

3 the bone

4   marrow. They become differentiated plasma

5 cells, and

6   the plasma cells secrete their antibodies. The

7   antibodies, as I already told you, aren't

8 secreted even

9   in an anamnestic response for a period of a few

10 days to

11   several days.

12   SPECIAL MASTER MILLMAN: So all of

13 this

14   process begins in a few days and extends over

15 how many

16   days or weeks?

17   THE WITNESS: Well, that's a very

18 interesting

19   question, and I think Dr. Bellanti tried to

20 address

21   some of this as well.

1   Now, remember, he used a term called

1   "homeostasis." We have to have some kind of

2   homeostatic mechanisms or built-in mechanisms to

3   control the darn response. Otherwise these

4 cells will

5   take off, proliferate, will be uncontrolled.

6 You'll

7   get a ton of antibodies, if -- and -- well, I'll

8 stop

9   there. So there's got to be some -- some

10 control. And

11   there is control that's mediated by a few

12 different

13   mechanisms.

14   You heard the term "T regulatory

15 cells"

16   mentioned yesterday. So one of the big breaks

17 on the

18   immune system are regulatory T cells. But also,

19 just

20   as -- just as MCD understanding is -- is moving

21 along,

1   well, an understanding of the complexities of

2   the

3   immune system is like growing in leaps and

4   bounds.   And

5   we know that there are other regulatory cells as

6   well,

7   not the least of which are B cells.   So it turns

8   out

9   that B cells also have the capacity to regulate

10 immune

11 responses, both physiologic responses and

12 autoimmune

13 responses.

14   So in the final case scenario, the --

15 the

16 acute effector cell response is controlled, but

17 that's

18 not to say that there aren't cells that are

19 still out

20 there that are capable of doing some of their

21 thing.

1   For instance, think about this for a second, we

2 get

3   immunized to -- and all of us should think about

4 this.

1   We get immunized to tetanus toxoid how often?

2 Once

3   every ten years. Well, that's amazing. Why do

4 we only

5   need to get immunized once every ten years?

6 Because it

7   turns out that those -- and the same is true for

8 other

9   vaccines, not necessarily ten years but five

10 years and

11   so forth.

12   Some -- the -- the -- it turns out

13 that when

14   the B cells differentiate the plasma cells,

15 which are

16   actually secreting the antibodies, protective

17   antibodies, that's why we get vaccinated, right,

18 that

19   they develop antibody secreting plasma cells,

20 but we

21   now know there's at least two populations of

1 antibody

2   screening plasma cells, some that are relatively

3 short

4   lived and others that are very long lived and

5 they hang

6   around for a long time --

7   SPECIAL MASTER MILLMAN: Ten years.

8   THE WITNESS: -- years to -- and where

9 -- and

10 they're capable of secreting antibodies.

11   And I'll just tell you one other thing

12 because the drug was mentioned today, and I'm

13 sure you

14 have some experience with this drug. And that's

15 Rituximab, a monoclonal antibody directed

16 against

17 B cells. And the thought was, well, not only is

18 that

19 drug, which was developed for B cell lymphoma, a

20 very

21 efficacious drug, but it turned out

1 serendipitously

1   that that drug was useful in some cases of B

2 cell or

3   auto antibody mediated diseases. Okay? But in

4 others,

5   it wasn't efficacious at all.

6   And the understanding is, at least

7 it's

8   believed to be due to the fact that there are

9 these

10   long lived -- there's this long-lived population

11 of

12   B cells that hangs out -- excuse me, long-lived

13   population of plasma cells that hangs out in the

14 bone

15   marrow that isn't touched by Rituximab. So they

16   continue to produce their auto antibody.

17   It's a little bit more complicated

18 than that,

19   but that's a long-winded answer to your

20 question.

21   SPECIAL MASTER MILLMAN: That's all

1 right.

2 Thank you.

3 Go ahead, Mr. Wishard.

4 MR. WISHARD: Thank you, ma'am.

5 BY MR. WISHARD:

6 Q. So, Dr. Levinson, we talked about your

7 views

8 on the innate immune system piece of this in

9 terms of

10 theory. The adaptive immune system piece of

11 this. I

12 think you also mentioned the cytokines.

13 And in terms of your review of the

14 records,

15 did JM have any -- after the October 1st, 2009,

16 vaccination, did he have any fever that you saw?

17 A. No.

1   Q.   Or myalgia or local vaccine site

2 reaction?

3   A.   No. And can I comment on that for a

4 second?

5   SPECIAL MASTER MILLMAN: Yes.

6   MR. WISHARD: Oh, sure.

7   THE WITNESS: Because you asked that

8 question

9   yesterday.

10   SPECIAL MASTER MILLMAN: Yes.

11   THE WITNESS: And that was a very

12 perceptive

13   question.

14   SPECIAL MASTER MILLMAN: Thank you.

15   THE WITNESS: Because innate immune

16 responses

17   which can be certainly manifested as a

18 consequence of

19   cytokines, like IL-6 which causes fever, IL-1

20 beta

21   which causes fever, when they are manifested

1   clinically, they are -- clinically. When

2 there's a lot

3   of cytokine involved, they're manifested by

4 myalgias,

5   muscle aches, arthralgias, joint aches, fevers,

6   headaches. And you would think -- I think you

7 would --

8   it would certainly be intuitive that if one were

9   developing a -- I don't want to put words in

10 anybody's

11   mouth -- a strong innate immune response that

12 was

13   reflected systemically to the point of these

14 factors

15   altering the function of epithelial podocytes,

16 that you

17   might have some of those symptoms. But in

18 addition,

19   this stuff is being injected into the muscle.

20 Patients

1   do get local reactions to injections, presumably

2   because of innate immune responses.

3   And we've not heard anything about JM

4   ever having had local or systemic kinds of

5 complaints

6   related to any of the vaccines that he received,

7   including the October flu vaccine.

8   SPECIAL MASTER MILLMAN: When you say

9   "local," you mean the left deltoid.

10   THE WITNESS: Yeah. Or wherever. I

11 mean --

12   SPECIAL MASTER MILLMAN: Well, I don't

13 know

14   where it was injected.

15   THE WITNESS: We don't know either.

16   SPECIAL MASTER MILLMAN: Yeah. Go

17 ahead.

18   BY MR. WISHARD:

19   Q.   During the questioning of Dr. Kaplan,

20 the

21   issue of steroids and how they work came up.

1 I'm going

2   to ask you to give a brief, in terms of your

3   understanding of that, because I think that you

4 have

5   some comments about that as well.

6   A.   Well, I have some comments about that,

7 but I

8   learned a fair amount about the -- the -- why

9 these,

10   quote/unquote, immunosuppressant agents are

11 useful in

12   treating MCD, or for that matter FSGS.   Until

13 this

14   proceeding or until this case came to my

15 attention, I

16   didn't know that immunosuppressive agents like

1   cyclosporin or even Rituximab or anti-

2 inflammatory

3   agents like corticosteroids, Prednisone,

4   methylprednisolone, which have some

5 immunosuppressive

6   effects that can block the action, steroids

7 block the

8   action of interleukin 2. They can reduce T cell

9   proliferation, and they can suppress clonal

10 expansion

11   of B cells in anaphylactic production. But

12 steroids

13   are not powerful immunosuppressants.

14   But the bottom -- the point I want to

15 try to

16   make is I didn't know that these agents had

17 these

18   off-target immune effects that are manifested in

19 the

20   treatment of a disease like MCD or FSGS. And I

21 was

1   bowled over by this. I have to tell you. And

2 so it's

3   true of a number of it -- what's it? That there

4 are

5   non-anti-inflammatory immunosuppressant effects

6 that

7   are meted out by a lot of these drugs that we

8 once

9   thought of only as immunosuppressive agents. So

10 that

11   includes agents that are used in MCD, steroids,

12   cyclosporin, calcineurin antagonist; inhibitors,

13   Rituximab, a beta set, something that didn't

14 come up

15   yet, mTOR inhibitors. These are all agents that

16   traditionally have been considered to be

17   immunosuppressive or anti-inflammatory agents

18 and were

19   used for that purpose, but turns out they've

20 been

21   harnessed for their use in a disease like MCD.

1 Because

1   why? Because they have direct effects on

2 podocyte

3   function, particularly on -- on preserving the

4 survival

5   of podocytes, stabilizing the podocyte foot

6 process

7   mechanism, the slit thing that you heard about,

8   stabilizing synaptopodin which I never heard

9 about

10   until today, a very important protein that's

11 involved

12   in podocyte function, stabilizing the actin

13   cytoskeleton framework of the podocytes, and I

14 could go

15   on and on.

16   And so to -- direct answer to your

17 question,

18   steroids have minor immunosuppressive activity.

19 They

20   have major anti-inflammatory activity. But

21 steroids

1   and this other category, class of agents that we

2 refer

3   to as immunosuppressive agents have direct

4 effects,

5   protective effects on the epithelial podocyte

6 foot

7   processes.

8   SPECIAL MASTER MILLMAN: So I think

9 what

10   you're saying is: That it seems to be

11 contradictory

12   that you would use an anti-inflammatory like

13 steroids,

14   Prednisone or Prograf, or immune-mediation

15 modulating

16   medicine on an illness that is neither

17 inflammatory or

18   immune mediated and, yet, they do help the

19 disease.

20   Is that what you're saying?

21   THE WITNESS: Well, I'm not sure I

1 would use

2   the word "contradictory," because as Dr.

3 Bellanti said,

1   this disease has undergone a -- a major

2   metamorphosis

3   in terms of our understanding of it, whereas it

4   used to

5   be thought to be predominantly an immune-

6   mediated

7   disease. That's why people reached -- put their

8   arms

9   out to the shelf to pull down steroids Prograf,

10   et cetera, et cetera, because they thought they

11   were

12   treating an immune-mediated disorder.

13   But lo and behold, as you heard Dr.

14   Kaplan

15   say, and I think Dr. Quan may have alluded to

16   this as

17   well, that turns out there's a whole new

18   understanding,

19   particularly from the molecular biological

20   understanding of podocytes and podocyte

21   function. So

1   it's not that it -- I don't think it's -- at

2 least I

3   don't think it's contradictory. I think it's

4   serendipitous that it was used and, lo and

5 behold, it

6   has direct -- a lot of these drugs have direct

7 effects

8   on podocyte function.

9   SPECIAL MASTER MILLMAN: I think of

10   serendipity as Pasteur seeing some virtue in

11 some mold

12   he didn't expect and from that, we get

13 penicillin. If

14   you don't like contradictory --

15   THE WITNESS: I didn't say I didn't

16 like it.

17   I said a word I'm not sure I would use.

18   SPECIAL MASTER MILLMAN: Oh, well,

19 let's

20   rephrase. Conundrum? Would you prefer

21 conundrum?

1 Mysterious?

2   THE WITNESS: No, I don't think it's a

3 conundrum now because I think we have a very

4 good

5 understanding at least of another -- another

6 manner,

7 another mechanism by which these drugs work.

8   SPECIAL MASTER MILLMAN: Okay.

9   THE WITNESS: That accounts for -- and

10 it at

11 least makes sense in terms of what people like

12 Dr. Kaplan and his colleagues have learned over

13 the

14 last decade, as he said, about the pathogenesis

15 of this

16 disease.

17   SPECIAL MASTER MILLMAN: It sounds

18 like a

19 bonus to the drug. A bonus no one anticipated,

20 but

21 they found it by serendipity. They gave

1 somebody this

2 thing -- I just heard on the radio, to interrupt

3 myself

4 there, that arsenic is used for childhood

5 leukemia. It

6 seems to be the only benefit. I don't know how

7 they

8 ever discovered that, but you would normally

9 expect

10 arsenic to be a poison. If you want to kill

11 somebody

12 on TV, you give them arsenic or something like

13 that.

14   THE WITNESS: Right.

15   SPECIAL MASTER MILLMAN: All right.

16 So how

17 did that -- how did that -- the radio did not

18 tell me

19 how they ever discovered that arsenic can treat

20 --

21 assuming this is true -- childhood leukemia.

1   THE WITNESS: That's because old lace

2   wouldn't work.

3   SPECIAL MASTER MILLMAN: What?

4   THE WITNESS: Old lace.

5   MR. WISHARD: Arsenic and Old Lace.

6   SPECIAL MASTER MILLMAN: Oh, right.

7   Wonderful picture.

8   Anyway, what I think you're saying is

9   that

10   because the concept of what minimal change

11   nephrotic

12   syndrome has changed from thinking it to be an

13   inflammatory disease, maybe immune mediated, and

14   then

15   recognizing it's neither, and yet when they use

16   steroids Prednisone, Prograf, which are

17   anti-inflammatory, or they use multiple immune

18   modulators all ending in "mab," that these work

19   and

20   they shouldn't work, but they do work, that

21   there's

1   a -- a -- something they don't know that's also

2   happening in these drugs which benefit the

3 podocytes

4   that are affected by minimal change nephrotic

5 syndrome.

6   Am I summing up what you said?

7   THE WITNESS: That's fine.

8   SPECIAL MASTER MILLMAN: You can

9 correct me.

10 You're the expert.

11   THE WITNESS: I would if I thought

12 needed,

13 but I don't think so here.

1   And let me just mention one other

2 thing about

3   it. There are papers that have been published

4 that

5   show -- and maybe Dr. Kaplan referred to this, I

6 don't

7   recall -- that show that cyclosporin works at

8 doses in

9   some patients that are considerably lower than

10 doses

11   that are needed to affect immunosuppression,

12 which goes

13   along with this whole notion -- that's more than

14 a

15   notion, but goes along with this whole new

16   understanding of how cyclosporin is working, and

17 it

18   certainly may be independent of its

19 immunosuppressive

20   activity.

21   SPECIAL MASTER MILLMAN: So, Doctor,

1 you

2   would not make the conclusion that because

3 Prednisone

4   or Prograf which are anti-inflammatory drugs and

5 other

6   drugs which are immune modulator drugs all

7 ending in

8   "mab" are used to treat minimal change nephrotic

9   syndrome; that, therefore, minimal change

10 nephrotic

11   syndrome is an anti -- is an -- excuse me, an

12   inflammatory disease or an immune-modulated

13 disease.

14   One does not lead to the other.

15   THE WITNESS: I better ask you to

16 repeat that

17   question.

18   SPECIAL MASTER MILLMAN: Yeah, yeah.

19   THE WITNESS: I'm sorry.

20   SPECIAL MASTER MILLMAN: I'll repeat

21 it for

694

1   you. It's in my brain. I'll just rewind it and

2 come

3   right back out.

4   You would not say that it was a fair

5   conclusion that just because doctors,

6 nephrologists,

7   continue to treat children with minimal change

8   nephrotic syndrome with Prednisone or Prograf

9 which are

10   anti-inflammatory or they may even resort to

11 drugs that

12   are immune modulators and all ending in "mab"

13 that

14   that, therefore, proves that minimal change

15 nephrotic

16   syndrome is an inflammatory disease or an

17   immune-mediated disease.

18   THE WITNESS: Absolutely I would not

19 say

20   that.

21   SPECIAL MASTER MILLMAN: All right.

1 Thank

2   you.

3   Go ahead, Mr. Wishard.

4   MR. WISHARD: Just a few additional

5   questions.

6 BY MR. WISHARD:

7   Q.   The issue of getting to the stroke

8 that

9   JM suffered from, the factor V Leiden issue.

10   Do you have additional thoughts? I

11 know

12 Dr. Kaplan had testified some about that as

13 well.

14   A.   So I have a thought about that. And

15 so my

16 thought now about that is more reflecting my

17 clinical

1   hat rather than a research hat. And I

2 understand based

3   on what I've heard from everybody in this room

4 that --

5   that has spoken on the issue, that thrombi are

6 unusual

7   in patients with MCD. Unusual. Particularly

8 kids,

9   yeah.

10   SPECIAL MASTER MILLMAN: Children.

11   THE WITNESS: Thank you. Thank you.

12 Kids.

13   And obviously -- and, unfortunately,

14 that was

15   a complication that JM experienced. And we've

16   heard about the likely, if not possible, role

17 that the

18   loss of anticlotting factors have in this whole

19   scenario. And you heard Dr. Kaplan talk about,

20 well,

21   what else could be going on? I mean, what else

1 doesn't

2   include the vaccine? I think we've ruled that

3 out

4   of -- of -- of everything, but everything

5 related to

6   the -- the MCD relapse.

7   And so when I am faced with a problem

8 like

9   this, I like to look at the entire picture and

10 look at

11   it holistically and try to think outside the box

12 and

13   consider any possibility that might -- might be

14   complicating the picture here.

15   And so as you've heard, it turns out

16 JM

17   has a factor V Leiden mutation. And as Dr. Quan

18   mentioned yesterday, well, gee, what effect does

19 that

20   have -- I'm paraphrasing now, what effect does

21 that

1   have? There are lots of normal folks who walk

2 around

3   with a factor V Leiden mutation, and they don't

4 have

5   any kinds of clots. So, again, I like to take a

6 step

7   back and try to look at the whole picture.

8   So we're faced with a situation now

9 where we

10   really don't understand why JM had these --

11   this -- these thrombotic episodes, and we're

12 searching

13   around for other factors. At least I say to

14 myself,

15   Well, wait a minute. JM isn't -- if you'll

16 pardon

17   the expression, JM, I'm sure you're a very

18 normal

19   guy in many respects, but at least at that time,

20 he

21   wasn't normal with regard to his health. He had

1 a risk

2 factor for developing thrombosis. And that was

3 he had

4 the nephrotic syndrome and proteinuria. He

5 didn't have

6 it as long as what Dr. Kaplan -- at least during

7 that

8 relapse, as long as what Dr. Kaplan would

9 consider long

10 enough to lose enough factors.

11   But wait a second. He's got this

12 factor V

13 Leiden abnormality which, as Dr. Kaplan pointed

14 out, is

15 not associated with bleeding as Dr. Bellanti

16 erroneously told us yesterday. It's associated

17 with

18 clotting, and I can explain why if anybody's

19 interested. So maybe it is a relevant factor.

20 It's

21 not that you can treat a factor V Leiden

1 abnormality of

2   this type, but maybe that's something that's

3 worth

1   considering.

2   Now, I'm not sitting here today and

3 saying

4   that that's what's going on here. But I think

5 it's

6   worth thinking about in terms of expanding the

7 box of

8   possibilities.

9   SPECIAL MASTER MILLMAN: Dr. Kaplan

10 didn't

11   say he wasn't excreting enough factors over that

12 period

13   of time. He wasn't excreting enough protein. I

14 don't

15   want to confuse factors with protein.

16   THE WITNESS: I'm sorry. What did you

17 say?

18   SPECIAL MASTER MILLMAN: I can repeat.

19 You

20   mentioned Dr. Kaplan had said he wasn't -- JM

21   wasn't excreting enough factors during the

1 period of

2   time that would lead to the CVA, and I think you

3 meant

4   protein, the protein, that anticlotting, pro

5 clotting

6   those factors.

7   THE WITNESS: Right, right, right.

8   SPECIAL MASTER MILLMAN: We all

9 misspeak

10   here. That's why we're helping each other.

11   Okay. Go ahead, Mr. Wishard.

12   MR. WISHARD: That's -- that concludes

13 my

14   direct examination.

15   SPECIAL MASTER MILLMAN: I don't know

16 if you

17   want to address this because this is a question

18 that

19   was asked of Dr. Kaplan and is appropriate for

20 him, but

1   I just thought I'd mention it, because Dr.

2 Bellanti

3   had -- I think it was Dr. Bellanti had said that

4 he

5   thought that everything that happened after

6   October 2nd, 2009, was just one long relapse.

7 And --

8   and not --

9   THE WITNESS: Yes.

10   SPECIAL MASTER MILLMAN: -- Dr. Kaplan

11 was

12   counting something like four or five --

13   THE WITNESS: Yes.

14   SPECIAL MASTER MILLMAN: -- since the

15   initial -- beginning of the disease, and then

16 the

17   relapse and then so on.

18   Did you want to weigh in on that?

19   THE WITNESS: I would defer to Dr.

20 Kaplan on

21   that. But I would say in response to that is I

1 don't

2 see -- he used the word, it's inconceivable that

3 the

4 vaccine per se led to the strokes that occurred

5 22 months down the road. I can't think of a way

6 that

7 one could explain that.

8   SPECIAL MASTER MILLMAN: It's hard to

9 explain

10 tort law to him. I can do it again if you want.

11 But

12 that's okay. You don't have to.

13   Thank you, Mr. Wishard.

14   Mr. McHugh, do you want to cross-

15 examine now

16 or do you want to have a break or what do you

17 want?

1   MR. McHUGH: Can we have 15 minutes?

2   SPECIAL MASTER MILLMAN: You want 15

3 minutes?

4   Okay. It's about 3:00 o'clock now. We'll break

5 and

6   we'll resume at 3:15. We'll go off the record

7 now.

8   Thank you.

9   (Whereupon a short recess was

10 taken.)

11   SPECIAL MASTER MILLMAN: All right.

12 Let's go

13 back on the record.

14   Mr. McHugh, would you like to do

15 cross-examination?

16   MR. McHUGH: Yes, Your Honor. I

17 appreciate

18 that.

19   SPECIAL MASTER MILLMAN: Go ahead.

20

21   CROSS-EXAMINATION

1   BY MR. McHUGH:

2   Q.   Doctor, good afternoon.

3   A.   Hello.

4   SPECIAL MASTER MILLMAN: And remember,

5   Mr. McHugh, you're going to have to speak up,

6 project,

7   because Dr. Levinson needs to be able to hear

8 you.   I

9   do too, actually.

10   MR. McHUGH: I get yelled at about

11 this all

12   the time.

13   /////

1   BY MR. McHUGH:

2   Q.   You seem to downplay the role of the

3   innate

4   immune system.

5   Is it not true that even some of the

6   adaptive

7   immune diseases, IGE, are finding an interplay

8   between

9   the innate and the adaptive systems?

10   A.   Well, we've known for a while that

11   there's an

12   interplay between the innate and adaptive

13   systems.

14   There's no question about that. But in this

15   case,

16   there is no adaptive immune response that I've

17   heard

18   anything about that could be related to the

19   immunopathogenesis of this young man's disease.

20   And in

21   addition, I haven't heard of any innate immune

1 response

2   that could be induced by -- as I explained

3 earlier,

4   that could be induced by an injection in the

5 skin into

6   the muscle that would lead to damage in the

7 podocyte.

8   I already told you, I think -- maybe I didn't

9 explain

10   it well. That's certainly possible -- that when

11 the

12   antigen is picked up and taken to the draining

13 lymph

14   node, there's an interaction in that lymph node

15 that

16   involves an innate immune response, not the

17 least of

18   which is the presentation of antigen by a cell

19 of the

20   innate immune system, i.e., a macrophage or

21 dendritic

1   cell. So yes, we've known for a long time that

2 there

3   is -- can be cross-talk between the innate and

4 adaptive

1   immune system, but I don't see how that plays a

2 role in

3   JM's disease.

4   Q.   You seem to indicate that because --

5   A.   Speak up, please.

6   Q.   Okay. You seem to indicate that

7 because the

8   injection is a distance from the kidney, that it

9 could

10   not affect the kidney.

11   How -- how long would it take for

12 something

13   injected in, say, the arm to reach the kidney?

14   A.   Well, I don't think the antigen

15 necessarily

16   reaches the kidney. I mean, I don't think

17 there's any

18   evidence that the antigen goes to the kidney and

19 is

20   removed by the kidney. That's not the -- the

21 mechanism

1   for removal of that antigen. It's destroyed by

2   --

3   ultimately by phagocytic cells. So I don't

4   think

5   that's relevant at all to this case.

6   Q.   I'm referring you to documents up on

7   the

8   screen. It should be on the screen in front of

9   you

10   there.

11   Can you tell us how you interpret

12   this?

13   A.   I haven't seen this paper, so ...

14   Q.   I can provide copies.

15   A.   If you'd like me to read the paper,

16   I'll be

17   happy to take a look at it.

18   MR. WISHARD: It's the Greenbaum

19   paper,

```
1    Exhibit --

2              SPECIAL MASTER MILLMAN:  Exhibit what?

3              MR. WISHARD:  He's the attorney,

4    please.

5              SPECIAL MASTER MILLMAN:  Exhibit what,

6    what?

7              MR. WISHARD:  It's the Greenbaum

8    paper,

9    Exhibit C at 17.

10             SPECIAL MASTER MILLMAN:  Seventeen.

11             MR. WISHARD:  Yes, ma'am.  I'm going

12   to give

13   him the whole paper.

14             SPECIAL MASTER MILLMAN:  Okay.  Thank

15   you.  I

16   have it.  Yes.  That's the one where you

17   eliminated

18   challenging the immune theory of the

19   pathogenesis of

20   childhood nephrotic syndrome in which disease is

21   caused
```

1   by T cells.

2   THE WITNESS: Okay. So I haven't read

3   through this paper in any critical or analytical

4   function. But if you want me to comment on what

5   I see

6   highlighted in yellow in this paragraph, I will

7   be

8   happy to say something about it. But I'll

9   reserve the

10   right to comment further on it once I've had a

11   chance

12   to sit down and read this paper in some

13   comprehensive

14   and critical fashion.

15   So what I'm seeing here, and I'll read

16   it,

17   "Although no single cytokine has been shown to

18   have a

19   direct causative role in nephrotic syndrome.

20   Several

1   studies have suggested a potentially important

2   role for

3   IL-13. For example, IL-13 expression was

4   reported to

5   be elevated in CD4 and CD8T cells in children

6   with

7   steroid sensitive nephrotic syndrome during a

8   relapse."

9   So the first question that I would

10   have to

11   ask is: When were these cells removed from

12   these

13   children with steroid sensitive nephrotic

14   syndrome?

15   Were they removed within a day of the

16   development of

17   the relapse? That's an important question.

18   Because

19   you're talking about a situation in -- or you're

20   --

21   your expert was talking about a situation in

1 which some

2 mysterious innate immune cytokine appears within

3 a

4 matter of short -- or cytokines appears within a

5 matter

6 of a few hours, or less than 18 hours, that

7 causes

8 damage to the kidney. So I don't know when

9 these cells

10 were taken.

11   And I would furthermore say that these

12 aren't

13 the only studies that reported on cytokines and,

14 in

15 particular, IL-13. So one of their earliest

16 studies

17 that was published, and I'm sure -- I'm pretty

18 sure it

19 was referred to in one of our reports, that

20 actually

21 planted the seed for factors or for permeability

1   factors being important in the pathogenesis of

2 MCD, is

3   a paper -- a famous paper that was published by

4   Shalhoub many years ago in which they talked

5 about a

1   permeability factor being secreted by

2 lymphocytes of

3   patients, T cells, by patients with MCD. Okay?

4   And it turns out, guess what, that if

5 you

6   mixed in certain cytokines to the in vitro

7 culture

8   system like IL-2, IL-12, and IL-15, those

9 cytokines

10   will lead to an increase in the production of

11 now a --

12   what was thought to be a permeability factor,

13   permeability of this podocyte filtering

14 mechanism, and

15   that factor production was inhibited by

16 cyclosporin and

17   corticosteroids.

18   But guess what, there were other

19 cytokines

20   that were added to those cultures which actually

21   decreased the production now of a permeability

1 factor.

2 We're not talking about IL-13 which may or may

3 not have

4 any permeability principles or functions. And

5 that's

6 not been looked at carefully. But guess what

7 happens?

8 If you put IL-13 and IL-4 into that culture

9 system, you

10 decrease the production of a permeability

11 factor. All

12 right?

13   So why am I telling you that? I'm

14 telling

15 you that because the studies are all over the

16 place,

17 and they have been all over the place for a

18 number of

19 years, so ...

20 BY MR. McHUGH:

21   Q. Is it true to say --

1   A.   So -- excuse me. Let me finish my

2 point.

3   So -- please.

4   So people have talked about cytokines

5 and

6   including IL-13, IL-14 as maybe being suggested

7 as a

8   potentially important item in the pathogenesis

9 of MCD.

10   But others have had contradictory results and

11 actually

12   show that they can decrease what had been

13 formerly

14   thought to be important permeability factors,

15 the

16   production of those permeability factors. And

17 it goes

18   on and on and on. And I think what some of the

19 experts

20   and, frankly, I'm not an expert in MCD, I'd like

21 to

1   think I know something about immunology, but the

2   experts in immunology and immunonephrology to

3 whom

4   Dr. Kaplan -- Kaplan, excuse me for pointing.

5 My

6   mother told me not to point -- when they think

7 about

8   this disease, in recent papers they talk about

9 the fact

10   that these factors are all over the place. Even

11 the

12   factors that have been shown to have what are

13 thought

14   to be permeability actions, permeability in the

15 kidney,

16   and they are measured by in vitro bioactivity

17 assays,

18   which are all over the place, not standardized,

19 they go

20   up, they go down in relationship to disease,

21 this -- or

1   not disease.   This one apparently happened to go

2 up in

3   terms of SSNS.   But they're all over the place.

4   And there are a number of factors that

5 have

1   been described not just cytokines, but all kinds

2   of

3   factors, hemopexin is probably the one that's

4   best

5   described and most studied. Has nothing to do

6   with the

7   immune system. Heparinex. It goes on and on

8   and on.

9   So my -- my first blush at this paper

10 doesn't

11 help me understand any better how cytokines like

12 IL-13

13 might be involved, but I will reserve final

14 judgment

15 until I read the paper.

16   Q.   Thank you.

17   MR. McHUGH: No further questions,

18 Your

19 Honor?

20   SPECIAL MASTER MILLMAN: Thank you.

21   Any redirect?

1   MR. WISHARD: No, ma'am.

2   SPECIAL MASTER MILLMAN: All right.

3 Are we

4   done with the testimony?

5   MR. WISHARD: Done with respondent's

6   testimony, yes, ma'am.

7   SPECIAL MASTER MILLMAN: And, Mr.

8 McHugh, I

9   assume. I had asked earlier. All right. Let's

10 --

11   let's do some housekeeping. Respondent is going

12 to

13   file Exhibit T when you get a chance.

14   MR. WISHARD: Yes, ma'am.

15   SPECIAL MASTER MILLMAN: And --

16   MR. WISHARD: This afternoon if I can.

1   SPECIAL MASTER MILLMAN: I'm sorry?

2   MR. WISHARD: By sometime this

3 afternoon if I

4 can.

5   SPECIAL MASTER MILLMAN: Okay. I hope

6 to get

7 an order out which will put in the things that I

8 would

9 like done.

10   And petitioner will file as Exhibit

11 101 which

12 is the video or whatever you call that was

13 screened

14 here for a few minutes. And then 102 to 107

15 would be

16 the articles that Dr. Bellanti and his Exhibit

17 100 had

18 put in a PowerPoint presentation, but you had

19 not filed

20 those articles.

21   MR. McHUGH: Right.

1   SPECIAL MASTER MILLMAN: Now, let me

2 ask:

3   Mr. Wishard, how much time would you like to be

4 able --

5   after Mr. McHugh files those articles to have

6   Dr. Kaplan and Dr. Levinson write reports, if

7 that's

8   sufficient? We are always open to having the

9   presumption of testimony. They can testify by

10 phone or

11   video camera. They don't have to traipse down

12 from

13   Pennsylvania. But if written reports are

14 sufficient

15   for you, how much time would you like to file

16 that?

17   MR. WISHARD: I don't -- I don't

18 anticipate

19   there will be any additional written reports;

20 however,

21   if I could have, once these articles are filed,

1 perhaps

1   20 days, 30 days just to make sure. I think

2 that we

3   have enough of an idea based upon the abstracts

4 that we

5   have from the articles, which we could pull up

6   ourselves. Some of them I could get for free,

7 some of

8   them I couldn't, but I do have I think maybe two

9 of the

10   eight physical articles in my possession, but

11 they

12   haven't been filed. Once they're filed, if I

13 could

14   have 20 to 30 days just to respond back and say,

15 We're

16   good to go, the record's closed, and respondent

17 would

18   move forward, and we're done.

19   SPECIAL MASTER MILLMAN: So in my

20 order, I'll

21   just say in 20 to 30 days -- I'll pick 30 days

1 because

2   you're going on vacation.

3   MR. WISHARD: Because I'm going to be

4 gone.

5   SPECIAL MASTER MILLMAN: Thirty days,

6 that's

7   right, unless you want to write it on vacation,

8 which I

9   don't think you do. In 30 days, you'll file a

10 status

11   report saying if you intend to file anything

12 further

13   from Dr. Kaplan and Dr. Levinson regarding the

14 new

15   Exhibits 1 to 107, you will. But if not, you

16 want to

17   just stay with the record.

18   MR. WISHARD: Yes, ma'am.

19   SPECIAL MASTER MILLMAN: Now, we have

20 two

21   alternative universes here. One is that the

1 record

2   will be closed. I don't know if you wanted to

3 do a

1   summation or waive. I don't know if you wanted

2 to do a

3   post-hearing brief or waive. Tell me what you

4 would

5   like to do, Mr. McHugh.

6   MR. McHUGH: I usually like to do

7   post-hearing briefs.

8   SPECIAL MASTER MILLMAN: So waive the

9   summation but do post hearing.

10   MR. McHUGH: Yep.

11   SPECIAL MASTER MILLMAN: Okay. Mr.

12 Wishard,

13   what would you like to do assuming we wrap up

14 sometime?

15   MR. WISHARD: I don't need to sum up

16 at this

17   point in time. I don't need to do post-hearing

18 briefs,

19   if Mr. McHugh is going to do one, I would like

20 the

21   opportunity.

1   SPECIAL MASTER MILLMAN: All right.

2 How long

3   after he files his post-hearing brief, would you

4 like

5   to file your post-hearing brief?

6   MR. WISHARD: Thirty days should be

7 fine.

8   And my response really is only what's come up

9 new in

10   this hearing, nothing in addition to what's

11 already

12   been said.

13   SPECIAL MASTER MILLMAN: All right.

14 If you

15   intend, Mr. McHugh, to file a reply to Mr.

16 Wishard's

17   response, how much time after he files his post-

18 hearing

19   brief would you like to file your reply, if you

20 file

1   one?

2   MR. McHUGH: One week.

3   SPECIAL MASTER MILLMAN: One week?

4   MR. McHUGH: One week.

5   SPECIAL MASTER MILLMAN: All right.

6 Seven

7   days.

8   Now, after the transcript comes in,

9 which I

10   think is what, three weeks, maybe, how much time

11 after

12   the transcript comes in, Mr. McHugh, would you

13 like to

14   file your post-hearing brief?

15   MR. McHUGH: One month.

16   SPECIAL MASTER MILLMAN: One month.

17 Okay.

18   Have I left out anything?   I don't

19 know.   I

20   don't think so.   No.

21   Well, I'd like to thank everybody for

1   persevering. It's hard to sit through almost

2 two days

3   of testimony, and it gets very technical. I

4 appreciate

5   the witnesses attending and coming in to do

6 that. And,

7   of course, Mr. Miles, Mrs. Miles, and their two

8   children.

9   MR. McHUGH: I do want to put Dr.

10 Bellanti

11   back.

12   SPECIAL MASTER MILLMAN: Oh, you want

13 to put

14   Dr. Bellanti on for rebuttal?

15   MR. McHUGH: Yes.

1   SPECIAL MASTER MILLMAN: How could I

2 have

3   forgotten this?   Okay.   Everybody sit down

4 except for

5   Mr. McHugh.

6   Dr. Bellanti, you'd like to take the

7 stand on

8   rebuttal.

9   Of course, Mr. Wishard, if you want to

10 have a

11   post rebuttal rebuttal, you can do that.   You'll

12 have

13   to consider what you want to do.

14   Remember if you're going to draw on

15 that --

16   what do we call that thing?   This paper.   We

17 have

18   paper.   It's a drawing board.   Then when you

19 talk, you

20   have to turn around and face the microphone.

21   All right.   Dr. Bellanti you're still

1 sworn

2 in, and Mr. McHugh hasn't asked you a question

3 yet, but

4 I guess you want to draw first.

5 Am I correct that you have drawn three

6 squares, and then you separated them into

7 sections? In

8 the upper left-hand corner you put "belief,"

9 underneath

10 it you put "faith," and you put belief, faith,

11 and next

12 to it you put "magic "--

13 THE WITNESS: Imagination.

14 SPECIAL MASTER MILLMAN: And

15 "imagination."

16 And what's under that? That's belief,

17 faith,

18 magic, and imagination and you're adding more in

19 red.

20 Ah-ha. What is that? In red you've

21 written

1   "medicine" and what?

2   THE WITNESS: "Research science."

3   SPECIAL MASTER MILLMAN: Research and

4   science, and you wanted to distinguish them on

5   all six

6   of those; is that correct?

7   THE WITNESS: That's correct.

8   SPECIAL MASTER MILLMAN: Okay. I

9   don't know

10   if you want Mr. McHugh to ask you a question or

11   just

12   you want to say -- what do you want to say,

13   Doctor?

14   What do you want to say, Mr. McHugh?

15

16   REBUTTAL EXAMINATION

17   BY MR. McHUGH:

18   Q.   I'd say please explain what you are

19   doing

20   there.

21   SPECIAL MASTER MILLMAN: But you have

1 to do

2   that in front of a microphone.

3   THE WITNESS: Well, thank you, Your

4 Honor,

5   for the opportunity to make some closing remarks

6 that

7   come to mind.

8   First of all, these two days have been

9 a -- a

10   very interesting and valuable experience for me,

11 and I

12   hope that the comments that we have given you

13 will help

14   you arrive at the truth.

15   I put --

1   MR. WISHARD: Special Master, Special

2   Master --

3   SPECIAL MASTER MILLMAN: Yes.

4   MR. WISHARD: -- I'm going to object

5 as this

6   is not proper rebuttal. The rebuttal should be

7 to

8   things that were brought up on --

9   SPECIAL MASTER MILLMAN: Oh, yes.

10   THE WITNESS: I'm coming to that.

11   MR. WISHARD: Well, can I finish my

12 question?

13   THE WITNESS: You finish.

14   MR. WISHARD: Thank you, sir.

15   My objection to this is: He's giving

16 a

17 closing argument. If he has specific questions

18 and

19 answers that Mr. McHugh wanted to provide to him

20 and

21 explain this chart that he prepared behind him,

1 that's

2   fine, and how it relates to what these two

3 gentlemen

4   testified to. But otherwise, I'm going to

5 object to

6   Dr. Bellanti giving a closing argument in this

7 case, in

8   addition to filing post-hearing briefs which

9   Mr. McHugh --

10   SPECIAL MASTER MILLMAN: Yes, I

11 understand.

12   What's that word after research?

13 What?

14   Research what?

15   THE WITNESS: Research science.

16   SPECIAL MASTER MILLMAN: Science.

1   THE WITNESS: Knowledge.

2   SPECIAL MASTER MILLMAN: All right.

3 Now,

4   what Mr. Wishard said is true, that rebuttal

5 should be

6   answers to questions pertaining to the testimony

7 of

8   opposing side's experts.   But we're a little

9 liberal

10   here.   So go ahead, say whatever it is you want

11 to say

12   that you put the one, two, three, four, five,

13 six,

14   seven -- no, eight -- two, four, six squares up

15 there.

16   Are we ending up in speculation?   Is

17 that

18   what magic is?   Imagination?

19 BY MR. McHUGH:

20   Q.   You have to answer the question.

21   SPECIAL MASTER MILLMAN: Sponge Bob

1 Square

2 Pants likes imagination.

3   THE WITNESS: Well, Your Honor, what

4 I'd like

5 to use this as an introduction to some of the

6 specific

7 comments that I'd like to direct to Dr. Kaplan

8 and

9 Dr. Levinson.

10   SPECIAL MASTER MILLMAN: Yes.

11   THE WITNESS: And I'd like to

12 introduce it

13 with the general concepts of how medicine should

14 --

15 proceeds and perhaps should proceed.

16   Medicine begins, as in ancient times,

17 with a

18 belief which in ancient civilizations had to do

19 with

20 faith. The medicine men and, of course, this

21 all

1   started with a belief or a faith. But we move

2 into the

3   second box where the belief/faith paradigm moves

4 to

5   magic and imagination. And some of the things,

6 and

7   unfortunately, we do it in medicine has a

8 certain magic

9   to it and certainly imagination. And of course,

10   Einstein said -- who's to quibble with Einstein.

11 He

12   said imagination is probably more important than

13   knowledge. You know, I'd leave it at that.

14   But -- but ultimately shown in red is

15   medicine, which is based on research and

16 knowledge and

17   science. And the evidence-based medicine is

18 what we

19   all try to do. And much of what I heard today

20 has less

21   of the medicine based on science and facts but

1 more

2 with the belief and more of an imagination that

3 I've

4 heard from both Dr. Kaplan and Dr. Levinson.

5 And to be specific, some of the things

6 that

7 Dr. Kaplan -- and I really appreciate his

8 erudite

9 beautiful presentation of his work and the

10 research

11 that he's done. But he -- he, unfortunately,

12 hobbles

13 around the belief. And he doesn't really get

14 into the

15 science. And specifically, he seems to downplay

16 the

17 role of infection and the relapse of nephrotic

18 syndrome. And I heard -- and I'm sure we heard

19 this

20 from Dr. Quan and from myself, and I can quote

21 the

1   literature that strongly supports a role of

2 infection,

1   particularly viral infection, that is involved

2 in the

3   relapse. And I think Dr. Kaplan seems to

4 downplay

5   that.

6   He also contradicts himself when he

7 first

8   says in testimony that he's sure that vaccines

9 do not

10   cause relapse. And then we see a video where he

11   specifically says that vaccines incur and

12 stimulate --

13   MR. WISHARD: Objection. That's not

14 what the

15   video said.

16   SPECIAL MASTER MILLMAN: Yeah, I know.

17 I've

18   heard it.

19   Look, we're all sitting in there.

20 It's a

21   2004 lecture based upon a 2003 article which is

1 ancient

2 history for nephrology at this point, and you

3 heard his

4 testimony.

5   THE WITNESS: Yes. Okay. And I

6 accept that,

7 Your Honor.

8   But the point is he minimizes the role

9 of

10 viral infection. Now --

11   SPECIAL MASTER MILLMAN: No. It's up

12 to me,

13 obviously, to believe whom I think is more

14 credible.

15 And when it comes to immunology, of course an

16 immunologist is going to be center. When it

17 comes to

18 nephrology, which is dealing with the kidneys,

19 it's

20 going to be a nephrologist and he's going to

21 know,

1   considering how much experience he's had, 5,000

2 times

3   more than you will.

4   THE WITNESS: That's right. And I

5 heard

6   Dr. Kaplan say that he would -- he's a

7 nephrologist. I

8   certainly accept that, but he's a pseudo

9 immunologist.

10   I'd like to be a immunologist and maybe a pseudo

11   nephrologist.

12   SPECIAL MASTER MILLMAN: Well, then

13 you're

14   both in the world of imagination. What can I

15 say?

16   THE WITNESS: At any rate, I do

17 appreciate

18   their -- their testimony. It's been very

19 erudite and

20   I've learned a lot. With regard to how an

21 infection, a

1   natural infection can relate to a vaccine-

2   induced

3   response, I've already commented on that from

4   the

5   Institute of Medicine. And they specifically

6   relate to

7   the relationship, that if something can occur in

8   a

9   viral infection, it can certainly form the basis

10 of a

11 vaccine.

12   SPECIAL MASTER MILLMAN: I have not

13 forgotten

14 your testimony, Doctor.

15   THE WITNESS: Now, with regard to

16 Dr. Levinson, he gave us a very erudite

17 discussion of

18 the adaptive immune response. And I completely

19 agree

20 with everything he said about the adaptive

21 response.

1   But in my testimony, as you indicated, Special

2 Master,

1   I focused on the role of the innate immune

2 system --

3   SPECIAL MASTER MILLMAN: You discussed

4 that.

5   THE WITNESS: -- injury. And Dr.

6 Levinson

7   seems to downplay that. He gave all kinds -- he

8   skirted around the issue.

9   SPECIAL MASTER MILLMAN: Well, you

10 disagree

11   with each other which is why we're sitting in a

12   courtroom.

13   THE WITNESS: I completely disagree,

14 and I

15   don't think that he takes into cognizance the

16 articles

17   that I referred to that referred to the Koenig

18 paper,

19   K-o-e-n-i-g --

20   SPECIAL MASTER MILLMAN: Yes. What

21   Mr. McHugh is going to provide us so we can all

1 get

2   educated.

3   THE WITNESS: I have them now and we

4 can

5   provide that.

6   -- that speak to the role of the

7 innate

8   system. All these other articles that relate to

9 IL-13,

10 Dr. Levinson seems to downplay that when you can

11 actually demonstrate IL-13, which is one of the

12 cytokines of the innate system deposited in the

13 glomerulus, I don't think you can give that

14 short

15 shrift.

16   So let's give him an opportunity to

17 review

1   the paper, and we can see what he says about it.

2   SPECIAL MASTER MILLMAN: Are you

3   finished?

4   THE WITNESS: He negates the -- in IGE

5   sensitivity, that we -- that you referred to

6   earlier,

7   which is not the case here, there is a definite

8   role of

9   the adaptive. We now know that the IGE that's

10   based on

11   cells of the innate system produce cytokines

12   that are

13   now receiving therapeutic attention in the

14   treatment of

15   these diseases, monoclonal antibodies, IL-13 to

16   4 to 5

17   that recruit eosinophils. So to give the innate

18   system

19   to short shrift, I think is not in keeping with

20   medicine based on science.

21   So the only comments other that I'd

1 like to

2   make is the paper by Greenbaum that was referred

3 to

4   earlier --

5   SPECIAL MASTER MILLMAN: Yes.

6   THE WITNESS: -- and Dr. Kaplan, you

7 know,

8   speaks to the points of how -- and I liked your

9   question by the way -- how can you not -- how do

10 you

11   explain a disease, minimal change disease, MCD,

12 that

13   has no inflammation and we're using drugs that

14 inhibit

15   inflammation?

16   SPECIAL MASTER MILLMAN: Dr. Levinson

17 --

18   THE WITNESS: The answer to that you

19 were

20   given is that perhaps there's some effect on

21 podocytes.

1   Well, that data is very shaky, and if you look

2   at the

3   Greenbaum paper --

4   MS. SOANES: May I ask what page of

5   the paper

6   you're quoting from --

7   THE WITNESS: I'm sorry?

8   MS. SOANES: -- so we can have that in

9   the

10   record.

11   MR. WISHARD: What page is this quote?

12   THE WITNESS: The Greenbaum paper is

13   on

14   page 446.

15   SPECIAL MASTER MILLMAN: It's C17,

16   just for

17   the record, and internal 446. This paper was

18   published

19   in 2012.

20   Are you on the right or the left of --

21   THE WITNESS: Yes.

1   SPECIAL MASTER MILLMAN: Which column

2 are you

3   in?

4   THE WITNESS: On page 446, first

5 column,

6   third paragraph, under "Currently available

7 treatments

8   oral glucocorticoids.   The efficacy of

9 glucocorticoids

10   in idiopathic nephrotic syndrome might be

11 attributable

12   to the immunosuppressive effects."   Or might --

13 or

14   there might be direct action on the podocytes.

15 So --

16   or possibly a combination of both.   So, you

17 know, it

18   isn't a black-and-white difference that we're

19 talking

1   about.

2   And the last point I would like to

3   make is,

4   several -- I think both Dr. Levinson and Kaplan

5   referred to as a dismissal of the T cell theory

6   that

7   once populated the literature with nephrotic

8   syndrome.

9   And I quite agree. It's not just the T cell.

10   That

11   theory has been pretty demolished, and these

12   other

13   theories that Dr. Kaplan mentioned are very

14   appropriate.

15   But I would like to suggest that the

16   data

17   involving the innate immune system with that

18   spectrum

19   of cytokines that are released in that early

20   response

21   explains the relapse of JM on October the 1st

1 when

2   he received the vaccine and the one-day relapse

3 that

4   ended up with proteinuria and a continuation of

5 that

6   process.

7   And the last slide I'd like to show is

8 that

9   other document from the -- from pharmacologic

10 and

11   medical device safety information report which

12   described some of the events that follow

13 injection of

14   an influenza vaccine that Dr. Levinson referred

15 to. He

16   was asking -- he was suggesting how could a

17 vaccine

18   that's been given in the muscle in the arm do

19 something

20   in the kidney?

21   Well, he even admitted that there are

1   sometimes cytokines that are produced. IL-1 for

2   example is the one that gives rise to this

3 fever. It

4   involves stimulation of the hypothalamus where

5 there is

6   the fever center. Other cytokines give rise to

7 the

8   aches.

9   Now, JM didn't have those responses

10   following his influenza, but there is -- there

11 are data

12   suggesting that cytokines from the innate system

13 are

14   responsible for some of the symptoms following

15 the

16   influenza vaccine.

17   I guess you don't need to show this --

18   MR. MILES: She's controlling it.

19   THE WITNESS: That's okay. We don't

20 need to

21   show that. It simply shows that following

1 injection of

2 the influenza vaccine with soreness, there is

3 the

4 documentation of the cytokines.

5 SPECIAL MASTER MILLMAN: But he didn't

6 have

7 any of those symptoms. You're saying that his

8 alleged

9 relapse is a symptom. He didn't have soreness

10 in his

11 arm. He didn't have swelling in his arm. He

12 didn't

13 have fever. He didn't have arthralgia. He

14 didn't have

15 myalgia. All he had was a relapse of his

16 minimal

17 change nephrotic syndrome. You're calling that

18 a

19 symptom of cytokine effect due to the vaccine.

20 THE WITNESS: When they do occur, but

21 I'm

1   saying that there could still be these factors

2 that

3   were in the belief, imagine -- imagination, and

4 these

5   permeability factors, I think many of those are

6   cytokines.

7   SPECIAL MASTER MILLMAN: I'm not going

8 into

9   magic or imagination or belief or faith because

10 I have

11   my marching orders to the federal circuit. I

12 don't

13   want to talk about legalities in front of all

14 these

15   people that aren't lawyers, but it requires that

16 I

17   find -- and I haven't ruled, obviously, but that

18 I find

19   a reasonable, prayerable, scientific, or medical

20 theory

21   explaining how flu vaccine can cause a relapse

1 of

2   minimal change nephrotic syndrome. Well, we

3 don't get

4   there yet.

5   If I find that, then I have to find

6 that it's

7   a logical sequence of cause and effect in this

8   particular case that it did do that.

9   And then the third thing I have to

10 find is

11   that the one day is an appropriate interval

12 between

13   vaccination and onset assuming I didn't find

14 onset

15   before the vaccination, and we're talking about

16   significant aggravation anyway, but one day is a

17   significant aggravation appropriate interval to

18 show

19   that the vaccine caused this relapse.

20   Those are all the three things I have

21 to

1   find, and none of it deals with belief, faith,

2 magic,

3   or imagination. So you can get rid of four of

4 those

5   six.

6   I forget to say to you, Mr. McHugh,

7 that I

8   had mentioned to you yesterday that when we were

9   following Exhibit 100, there were many pages,

10 shall we

11   call them pages, which were screened in the

12 PowerPoint

13   that we didn't have, and they were showing

14   progressions. This happens, then something

15 else, and

16   it was a little confusing and there's an awful

17 lot of

18   repetition in 100. You might take out

19 repetitive

20   pages. Just go over it. You've got the time.

21 You've

1   got 30 days.

2   THE WITNESS: I resubmitted that, Your

3   Honor,

4   in the form that I gave it so you would be able

5   -- if

6   you receive a live -- I mean, a -- an electronic

7   version, you can play it and show the --

8   SPECIAL MASTER MILLMAN: Not

9   happening.

10 So --

11   THE WITNESS: You will have it.

12   SPECIAL MASTER MILLMAN: -- just

13 figure out

14 for yourself, Mr. McHugh. You know, a lazy

15 Sunday

16 afternoon, your grandchildren will be asleep,

17 and you

18 can figure out, How can I help the special

19 master

20 understand in hard copy form what it is that

21 transpired

1   during the PowerPoint presentation?

2   MR. McHUGH: I'll get that done.

3   SPECIAL MASTER MILLMAN: You can mark

4 that as

5   Exhibit 108 if you like.

6   MR. McHUGH: I just have one more

7 question.

8   SPECIAL MASTER MILLMAN: Yes. Go

9 right

10   ahead.

11   BY MR. McHUGH:

12   Q.   Doctor, in reading the Greenbaum

13 article, do

14   you agree that that article basically eliminates

15 the

16   idea that this is -- there's an immune factor

17 here?

18   SPECIAL MASTER MILLMAN: That this is

19 a what?

20   BY MR. McHUGH:

21   Q.   Eliminate the idea -- doctors have

1 basically

2   held that they treat this thing with the

3 steroids

4   because of -- of the -- it's an immune -- it --

5 it cuts

6   down the immune system effect. And they think

7 that's

8   involved in nephrotic syndrome.

9   A.   I do.

10   Q.   Does the Greenbaum article eliminate

11 that as

12   a possibility or does it come up with something?

13   SPECIAL MASTER MILLMAN: I don't think

14 that's

15   what it says. At the end of it which is page --

16   internal page 454, I'm looking at C17 because

17   respondent filed it as an exhibit, "The

18 recognition of

1   the crucial role of podocyte" -- podocyte --

2 "podocyte

3   injury in nephrotic syndrome has led to many new

4   studies that have identified several important

5   molecular pathways that are able to regulate

6 podocyte

7   injury," which suggests to me why the first page

8   abstract has in the next to last, if you like

9 the word

10   "penultimate", sentence, "challenging the immune

11 theory

12   'so the pathogenesis of childhood nephrotic

13 syndrome in

14   which diseases caused by T cells.'"

15   This is suggesting to me that, as Dr.

16 Kaplan

17   testified, the concept of what exactly minimal

18 change

19   nephrotic syndrome is has changed over the last

20 ten

21   years, and that this article which was written

1 in 2012

2   is in the middle of those ten years. And so

3 we're not

4   now, according to Dr. Kaplan, in the world of

5   inflammatory disease or immune-mediated disease

6 even

7   though the treatments, the steroids, the

8   anti-inflammatory, Prednisone and Prograf, and

9 the

10   immune modulators all ending in "mab" are still

11 used,

12   but not because they have an effect on an

13 illness

14   that's not inflammatory or immune mediated, but

15 because

16   there's some other beneficial factor which helps

17 the

18   person who -- the child who has minimal change

19   nephrotic syndrome.

20   I hope I've summarized that correctly.

1   Everybody nod their head.

2   THE WITNESS: Yes. I think the

3 article

4   dismisses the old theory that I think Dr. Kaplan

5 and --

6   and Special Master are referring to, that it's T

7 cell

8   driven. That was a prevalent theory, I don't

9 know, 10,

10   15 years ago, but that's been dismissed.

11   I think the new data is suggesting the

12 role

13   of the innate system, and several of the

14 articles that

15   I submitted speak to that point. So some of

16 these

17   factors, these belief, faith factors, may be

18 based on

19   that data related to factors that have come from

20 the

21   innate system.

1   SPECIAL MASTER MILLMAN: I will tell

2 you that

3   I haven't memorized all these articles.   There's

4 lots

5   of them and they're very technical, but I will

6 be

7   skeptical about an article that deals with an

8 adult who

9   has minimal change disease or nephrotic syndrome

10   because of what Dr. Quan said, it's a totally

11 different

12   disease in an adult than in a child.

13   THE WITNESS: Yes, yes.

14   SPECIAL MASTER MILLMAN: And No. 2, if

15   they're old.   If they predate 2007, I'm going to

16 say,

17   well, you know, if their understanding is

18 they're

19   dealing with an inflammatory disease or they're

20 dealing

21   with an immune-modulated disease, because we

1 know

1   steroids work or whatever they were giving for

2   immune-mediated diseases, then I'm going to

3 think

4   about, well, you know, how credible is that now?

5 If --

6   if the science, which I did not invent, if the

7 science

8   is changing, if the understanding by people who

9 are

10   versed in this, which I am not, if the people

11 upon who

12   I'm supposed to rely are saying the concept of

13 this

14   disease is changing, then I have to bow to that.

15 I am

16   bowing to experts. So there we have it.

17   Did you have any more questions?

18   MR. McHUGH: No, Your Honor, I'm done.

19   SPECIAL MASTER MILLMAN: Thank you

20 very much,

21   Dr. Bellanti.

1   Thank you, Mr. McHugh.

2   Did you want to put on any of --

3 either of

4 your two witnesses, Dr. Kaplan or --

5   MR. WISHARD: No, ma'am.

6   SPECIAL MASTER MILLMAN: No? Are we

7 done?

8 Are we going off the record now.

9   MR. WISHARD: Absolutely.

10   SPECIAL MASTER MILLMAN: All right.

11 Thank

12 you very much again. I appreciate your

13 participation.

14 Thank you. We'll go off the record now.

15   (The proceedings were

16   concluded at 3:56 p.m.)

1   CERTIFICATE OF TRANSCRIBER

2

3   I, Kristy L. Clark, court-approved

4 transcriber,

5   certify that the foregoing is a correct

6 transcript from the

7   official electronic sound recording of the

8 proceedings in the

9   above-titled matter.

10

11

12

13   DATE: 11/8/17

14   KRISTY L. CLARK

15

16

17

18

19

20

21 **END OF TRANSCRIPT:**

1

2 Notes from Author

3

4 THIS IS THE OFFICIAL TRANSCRIPT OF DAY TWO OF THE

5 MILES V. SECRETARY ALEX AZAR, DEPARTMENT OF HEALTH

6 AND HUMAN SERVICES' VACCINE INJURY COMPENSATION

7 PROGRAM TRIAL.

8

9 ALL SPELLING AND GRAMMATICAL ERRORS ARE FROM THE

10 GOVERNMENT'S TRANSCRIBER.

11

12 FOR FURTHER DETAILS AND COMMENTARY BY MR. MILES,

13 PLEASE GO TO PETITIONER'S

14 TRANSCRIPT VERSION OF TRIAL. ALSO AVAILABLE ON

15 AMAZON AS A COMPANION BOOK.

16

17 WHERE THE PETITIONER WILL ATTEMPY TO EXPLAIN THE

18 SCIENCE, THE ADVERSE VACCINE REACTION, AND THE

19 GENERAL FOOLISHNESS OF THE VACCINE INJURY

20 COMPNSATION PROGRAM AND GOVERNMENT EXPERTS.

21

1 IT IS A HIGHLY FOOLISH PROGRAM, CREATED BY A

2 HIGHLY FOOLISH VACCINE ACT ENACTED IN 1986.

3

4 ALL CITZENS SHOULD BECOME FAMILIAR WITH THE LAW

5 AND ALL VACCINE-RELATED PROGRAMS, BEFORE BEING

6 VACCINATED. I RECOMMEND VNTY,VACCINE NO THANK

7 YOU, AS MY ANSWER TO INFLUENZA AND COVID. THESE

8 VACCINES HAVE POOR SAFETY PROFILES, AND ZERO

9 LAIBILITY AGAINST VACCINE MANUFACTURES AND MEDICAL

10 PROFESSIONALS.

11

12 I BELIEVE MOST CITIZENS DO NOT NEED THESE

13 VOLUNTARY VACCINES, AND I REJECT THESE VACCINES

14 SPECIFICALLY AS A PROPER PROTECTION TOOL. AS

15 BETTER THERAPEUTIC PROTOCOLS EXIST.

16

17 AS ALWAYS, IT IS A CITIZENS RIGHT TO CHOOSE WHAT

18 WORKS BEST FOR THEM AND THEIR LOVED ONES BUT

19 BEWARE OF A FALSE PROMISES BY OUR GOVERNMENT AND A

20 VICP PROGRAM LURKING IN THE BACKGROUND IF A

21 CITIZEN DEVELOPS AN ADVERSE VACCINE REACTION.

1 THERE IS NO SAFETY NET.

2

3

4

5

6

7

8 # FAIR

9 # WARNING

www.ingramcontent.com/pod-product-compliance
Lightning Source LLC
Chambersburg PA
CBHW062045270326
41931CB00013B/2948